Lasers in dentistry

Lasers in dentistry

S Parker
BDS, LDS RCS, MFGDP
Dental Surgeon
30 East Parade
Harrogate
North Yorkshire
HG1 5LT

thewholetooth@easynet.co.uk

2007
Published by the British Dental Association
64 Wimpole Street, London, W1G 8YS, UK

Foreword

"Lasers are just looking for a home in dentistry"

Such comment sought to refute the introduction of the first dental laser in 1989. In the brief period that has elapsed since then, laser use has been shown to be of benefit in all aspects of clinical dental practice.

Research undertaken at major institutions around the world has established the scientific and evidence base of laser light interaction with all oral tissue and has provided confidence to those who seek to employ the broad array of laser wavelengths as an adjunct to their provision of dental care.

I am indebted to Dr Terry Myers for his personal encouragement in 1989. His dream to see laser light transform dentistry has encouraged many and has certainly changed my professional life.

I acknowledge my friends at the Academy of Laser Dentistry whose insight, support and encouragement gave me the opportunity to develop my interest in lasers, together with my wife, Penny whose forbearance has allowed me to undertake this review.

I hope you will enjoy this book. It is as much the result of my own quest for answers as it is a representation of research, anecdote and clinical procedures with lasers. I hope it may provide greater understanding of this exciting treatment modality.

Steven Parker
Harrogate
October 2007

2007

Published by British Dental Journal Books

© 2007

All rights reserved. No part of this publication may be reproduced stored in a retrieval system, or transmitted in any form or by any means electronic, mechanical, photocopying, recording or otherwise, without either the permission of the publisher or a licence permitting restricted copying in the United Kingdom issues by the Copyright Licensing Agency Limited,
90 Tottenham Court Road, London WC1 9HE

ISBN 978 0 904588 95 8

Printed and bound by
Dennis Barber Limited. Lowestoft, Suffolk

Contents

Introduction, history of lasers and laser light production	1
Laser-tissue interaction	12
Low-level laser use in dentistry	21
Lasers and soft tissue: 'loose' soft tissue surgery	29
Lasers and soft tissue: 'fixed' soft tissue surgery	36
Lasers and soft tissue: periodontal therapy	43
Surgical laser use in implantology and endodontics	50
Surgical lasers and hard dental tissue	60
Laser regulation and safety in general dental practice	70
Index	80

IN BRIEF

- 'Laser' is an acronym for 'light amplification by the stimulation emission of radiation'. Its theoretical basis was postulated by Albert Einstein.
- The first tooth exposed to laser light was in 1960.
- Lasers can be applied to almost any clinical situation.
- Laser light in dentistry is a unique, non-ionising form of electromagnetic radiation that can be employed as a controlled source of tissue stimulation, cutting or ablation, depending on specific parameters of wavelength, power and target tissue.

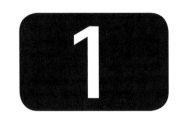

Introduction, history of lasers and laser light production

The word laser conjures in the mind's eye many aspects of what might be described as 'modern' life. The words 'powerful', 'precise' and 'innovative' complement our conception of the world in terms of technology, whereas patients often associate the words 'magical' and 'lightening quick' with the use of lasers in medical practice. The purpose of this book is to explore the history and development of lasers, the integration of lasers into clinical dentistry and the safeguards as to their regulated use.

LASERS IN DENTISTRY

1. Introduction, history of lasers and laser light production
2. Laser-tissue interaction
3. Low-level laser use in dentistry
4. Lasers and soft tissue: 'loose' soft tissue surgery
5. Lasers and soft tissue: 'fixed' soft tissue surgery
6. Lasers and soft tissue: periodontal therapy
7. Surgical laser use in implantology and endodontics
8. Surgical lasers and hard dental tissue
9. Laser regulation and safety in general dental practice

INTRODUCTION

The theoretical basis of laser light production was developed some 90 years ago; the first laser was used on an extracted tooth 47 years ago. It is perhaps somewhat surprising that commercially available lasers have only been used in dental practice during the past 18 years. Associated with the launch of the first 'dental' laser, there was a level of hype that quickly led to a combination of frustration for dentists and research that discredited or minimised many of the claims for clinical use (Fig. 1).

Unlike many fields of medicine and surgery, where laser treatment represents a sole source of remedy, in dentistry the use of a laser is considered adjunctive in delivering a stage of tissue management conducive to achieving a completed hard or soft tissue procedure.

To the dental professional in general practice, the delivery of dental treatment can be compromised by the willingness of the patient to accept a procedure that is often erroneously associated with painful stimuli. Most patients recoil at the thought of a high or low-speed drill and those exposed to surgery find associated bleeding and tissue bruising interferes with normal speech and eating functions. As much as any wish to explore the envelope of possible laser-tissue interaction, much of the hype surrounding laser use in dentistry has centred on the possibility to encourage patient uptake through the avoidance of peri- and post-operative pain and discomfort. Certainly, however, today's lasers offer an opportunity to deliver hard and soft-tissue treatments that, at least in outline, make the patient experience somewhat easier (Figs 2-10).

As will be seen in later chapters in this book, considerable research has been carried out ostensibly to validate the innovative use of lasers in all branches of dentistry. At worst, claims to beneficial use in some areas have been discredited; often, other usage has been shown to overcome deficiencies in more conventional therapies. Lasers can be applied to almost any clinical situation, but their efficacy *versus* conventional techniques in many cases is unknown, with the exception of anecdotal reports.

Essentially, the adjunctive use of surgical lasers in dentistry has sought to address efficient cutting of dental hard tissue, haemostatic ablation of soft tissue and also the sterilising effect through bacterial elimination. Less powerful, non-surgical lasers have been shown to modify cellular activity and enhance biochemical pathways associated with tissue healing, aid in caries detection and assist in the curing of composite restorative materials. The decision to include lasers in everyday dental care will depend not least upon financial considerations as to how their

LASERS IN DENTISTRY

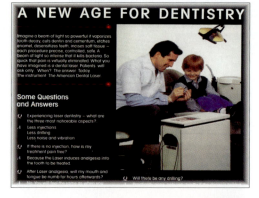

Fig. 1 An example of the promotional material available for patient motivation, printed in 1990. The laser wavelength being described (Nd:YAG) is almost exclusively for soft tissue procedures

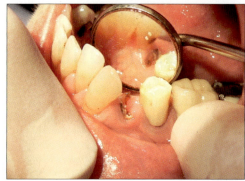

Fig. 2 Pre-operative view of fractured tooth with gingival overgrowth on to root surface

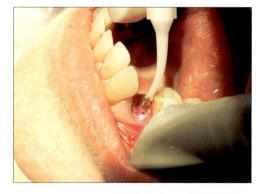

Fig. 3 Diode laser used to remove excess soft tissue

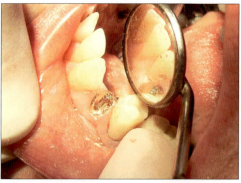

Fig. 4 Immediate post-laser treatment, with post retention for core material

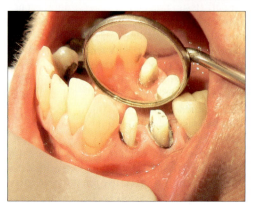

Fig. 5 Healing at one week

use may enhance practice profitability; the greatest factor in making that decision will be an understanding of how laser wavelengths interact with oral tissue, together with an appreciation of how such use can improve patient management.

HISTORY OF LASERS AND THEIR USE IN CLINICAL MEDICINE AND DENTISTRY

The theoretical basis that postulated the production of intense light of a specific configuration, pre-dated the development of the first laser by over forty years.

In 1704, Newton[1] characterised light as a stream of particles. The Young's interference experiment in 1803 and the discovery of the polarity of light convinced other scientists of that time that light was emitted in the form of waves. The concept of electromagnetic radiation, of which 'light' is an example, had been described in mathematical form by Maxwell, in 1880. Maxwell's electromagnetic (EM) theory explained light as rapid vibrations of EM fields due to the oscillation of charged particles. At the turn of the 20th century, the black body radiation phenomenon challenged the waveform light theory. Atomic structures would absorb incident EM energy and become excited to an upper level, which would subsequently decay to a lower, stable state, with the release of emissive energy. According to Maxwell's EM theory, the energy intensity of EM emissions with a given frequency is proportional to the square of this frequency.

Additional work undertaken by Hertz on the 'photoelectric effect' (a pioneering study into cathode ray emission), and Planck on the formulation of the distribution of the radiation emitted by a black body or perfect absorber of radiant energy, complemented further the understanding of light propagation. The significance of Planck's constant in this context is that radiation such as light, is emitted, transmitted and absorbed in discrete energy packets or quanta, determined by the frequency of the radiation and the value of Planck's constant.

The observations that the number of electrons released in the photoelectric effect is proportional to the intensity of the light and that the frequency, or wavelength, of light determines the maximum kinetic energy of the electrons, indicated a kind of interaction between light and matter that could not be explained in terms of classical physics. The search for an explanation led in 1905 to Albert Einstein's fundamental theory that light can be regarded alternatively as composed of discrete particles (photons), equivalent to energy quanta.

In explaining the photoelectric effect, Einstein (Fig. 11) assumed that a photon could penetrate matter, where it would collide with an atom. Since all atoms have electrons, an electron would be ejected from the atom by the energy of the photon, with great velocity.

INTRODUCTION

Einstein also predicted in 1917 in *Zur Theorie der Strahlung*[2] (Theory of Wavelength), that when there exists the population inversion between the upper and lower energy levels among the atom systems, it was possible to realise amplified stimulated radiation, ie laser light. Stimulated electromagnetic radiation emission has the same frequency (wavelength) and phase (coherence) as the incident radiation.

MASER

The electromagnetic spectrum is a comparative arrangement of electromagnetic energy (photonic quanta) relative to wavelength, spanning ultra-short gamma and X-radiation, through visible light, to ultra-long micro- and radio-waves. In 1953, Charles Townes, experimenting with microwaves,[3] produced a device whereby this radiation could be amplified by passing it through ammonia gas. This was the first MASER (microwave amplification by the stimulated emission of radiation) and was developed as an aid to communication systems and time-keeping (the 'atomic clock'). It was realised that only a fraction of the incident energy was converted into maser energy, the greater emission being in the form of heat; the output power of the early masers was of the order of a few micro-watts.

Experimental work undertaken by other workers into various incident energy wavelengths and target materials, resulted in the invention of the first LASER (light amplification by the stimulated emission of radiation) by Theodore Maiman,[4] at the Hughes Aircraft Company USA, in 1960.

LASER

The experimental work into the physics of laser light production highlighted the attraction of the use of intense radiation energy, of single wavelength, in many military and communications applications. Maiman's laser used a solid ruby as an 'active medium', which was energised or 'pumped' by an electrical source (Fig. 12).

Many other kinds of laser were invented soon after the solid ruby laser – the first uranium laser by IBM Laboratories (in November 1960), the first helium-neon laser by Bell Laboratories in 1961 and the first semiconductor laser by Robert Hall at General Electric Laboratories in 1962; the first working neodymium-doped yttrium aluminium garnet (Nd:YAG) laser and CO_2 laser by Bell Laboratories in 1964, argon ion laser in 1964, chemical laser in 1965 and metal vapour laser in 1966. In each case, the 'name' of the laser was annotated with regard to the active medium (source of laser photons) used.

Laser use in medicine and surgery

As will be seen in later chapters, there is a specific and fundamental relationship between light wavelength and absorption by an 'illuminated' target material. Thus, the unique nature

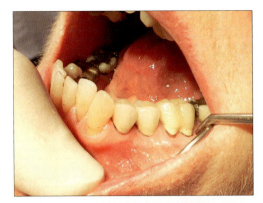

Fig. 6 Final restorations fitted

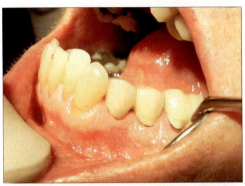

Fig. 7 Situation at one year. Note stability of gingival margins

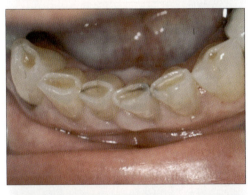

Fig. 8 Abrasion cavities, lower incisors

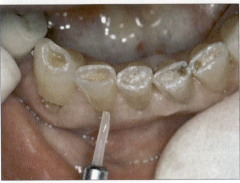

Fig. 9 Use of erbium laser to define cavity extent and condition of hard tissue prior to etching and restoration

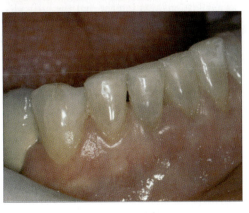

Fig. 10 Completed restorations

LASERS IN DENTISTRY

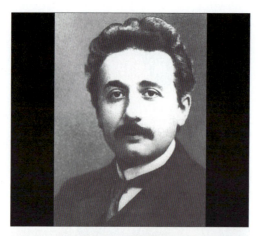

Fig. 11 Albert Einstein, 1879–1955

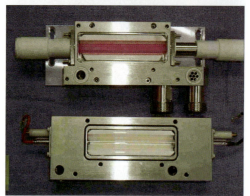

Fig. 12 Example of a ruby rod active medium, similar to that used in Maiman's first laser

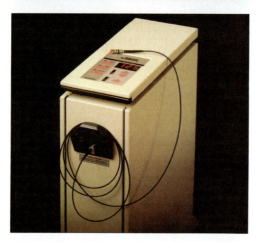

Fig. 13 DLase 300 Nd:YAG laser (American Dental Technologies)

of laser light and its specific absorption, led to an expansion of its use in medicine. Within a year of the invention, pioneers such as Dr Leon Goldman began research on the interaction of laser light on biologic systems, including early clinical studies on humans.[5] Interest in medical applications was intense, but the difficulty controlling the power output and delivery of laser energy, together with the relatively poor absorption of these red and infrared wavelengths, led to inconsistent and disappointing results in early experiments. The exception was the application of the ruby laser in retinal surgery in the mid-1960s. In 1964, the argon ion laser was developed. This continuous wave 488 nm (blue-green) gas laser was easy to control and its high absorption by haemoglobin made it well suited to retinal surgery; clinical systems for treatment of retinal diseases were soon available.

In 1964, the Nd:YAG and CO_2 lasers were developed at Bell Laboratories in the USA. The CO_2 laser is a continuous wave gas laser and emits infrared light at 10,600 nm in an easily manipulated, focused beam that is well absorbed by water. Because soft tissue consists mostly of water, researchers found that a CO_2 laser beam could cut tissue like a scalpel, but with minimal blood loss. The surgical uses of this laser were investigated extensively from 1967-1970 by pioneers such as Dr Thomas Polanyi and Geza Jako and in the early 1970s, use of the CO_2 laser in ENT and gynaecologic surgery became well established, but was limited to academic and teaching hospitals.

In the early 1980s, smaller but more powerful lasers became available. Most of these systems were CO_2 lasers used for cutting and vaporising tissue and argon lasers for ophthalmic use. These 'second generation' lasers were all continuous wave or CW systems which tend to cause non-selective heat injury, and proper use required a long 'learning curve' and experienced laser surgeons.

The single most significant advance in the use of medical lasers was the concept of 'pulsing' the laser beam, which allowed selective destruction of abnormal or diseased tissue, while leaving surrounding normal tissue undisturbed. The first lasers to fully exploit this principal of 'selective thermolysis' were the pulsed dye lasers introduced in the late 1980s for the treatment of port wine stains in children and shortly after, the first 'Q-switched' (ultra-short pulsed) lasers for the treatment of tattoos. Another major advance was the introduction of scanning devices in the early 1990s, enabling precision computerised control of laser beams. Scanned, pulsed lasers revolutionised the practice of plastic and cosmetic surgery by making safe, consistent laser re-surfacing possible, as well as increasing public awareness of laser medicine and surgery.

Laser use in dentistry

Although Maiman had exposed an extracted tooth to his ruby laser in 1960, the possibilities for laser use in dentistry did not occur until 1989, with the production of the American Dental Laser for commercial use. This laser, using an active medium of Nd:YAG, emitted pulsed light and was developed and marketed by Dr Terry Myers, an American dentist. Though low-powered and due to its emission wavelength, inappropriate for use on dental hard tissue,[6] the availability of a dedicated laser for oral use gained popularity amongst dentists. This laser was first sold in the UK in 1990 (Fig. 13).

Other laser wavelengths, using machines that were already in use in medicine and surgery and only slightly modified, became available for dental use in the early 1990s. Being predominately argon, Nd:YAG, CO_2 and

INTRODUCTION

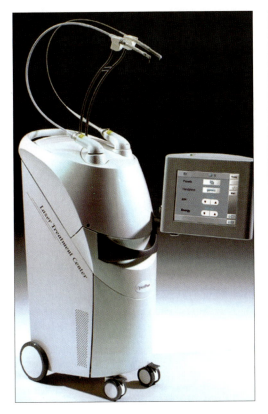
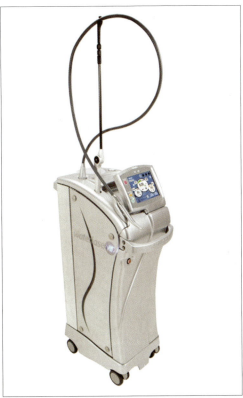

Figs 14 and 15 Examples of modern surgical dental lasers: combined Er:YAG/CO_2 (Fig. 14, left) and Nd:YAG (Fig. 15, right)

semiconductor diodes, all these lasers failed to address a growing need amongst dentists and patients for a laser that would ablate dental hard tissue. In 1989, experimental work by Keller and Hibst[7] using a pulsed erbium YAG (2,940 nm) laser, demonstrated its effectiveness in cutting enamel, dentine and bone. This laser became commercially available in the UK in 1995 and, shortly followed by a similar Er,Cr:YSGG (erbium chromium: yttrium scandium gallium garnet) laser in 1997, amounted to a laser armamentarium that would address the surgical needs of clinical dentistry in general practice (Figs 14 and 15).

LIGHT (PHOTONIC) PRODUCTION AND EMISSION
Ordinary light

'Ordinary' light refers to the close band of wavelengths in the electromagnetic spectrum that is visible to the human retina. In nature, its origin is in the cosmic stream from space and a common source of man-made ordinary light is the incandescent filament of a light bulb. 'White' light is the sum of all component wavelengths of the visual spectrum. The waveform of ordinary light is non-coherent, in that there is a confused overlap of successive waves. The spread of such waves results in scattering of light with distance and the multi-direction and interference of successive waves gives rise to divergence and dimming with distance. The wavelength of any light beam is measured in metres, with typical values being expressed as nanometres (10^{-9} metres).

The unit of light energy is the photon and the relationship of energy with frequency can be expressed as:

$$E = h\nu$$

where ν = frequency (number of wave oscillations with time) and h = Planck's constant.

In addition, the relationship of frequency to wavelength λ can be expressed as:
$$c = \nu \div \lambda$$
where c is the speed of light (a constant).

Substituting wavelength for frequency:
$$E = (hc) \div \lambda$$

This relationship thereby establishes an inverse relationship between wavelength and photonic energy. With reference to the electromagnetic spectrum, this accounts for why X-rays, at the ultra-short wavelength end of the spectrum have deep penetrating energy, whilst long wavelength radio waves require a specific receiver.

Quantum nature of light – absorption & emission

The expression of quantum physics in terms of atomic structure was defined by Bohr in 1922.[8] Incident light energy, absorbed by a target atom, will result in an electron moving to a higher energy shell. This unstable state will result in the emission of photonic energy relative to the stable energy state of the target, with excess energy being produced as heat. This is known as spontaneous emission. If an already energised atom is bombarded with a second photon, this will result in the emission of two, coherent photons of identical wavelength. This was postulated by Einstein as stimulated emission[2] (Fig. 16).

The simple process represented by Figure 16 demonstrates a three-level concept of energy

LASERS IN DENTISTRY

Fig. 16 Photonic emission, showing spontaneous (Bohr's model, upper) and stimulated emission (Einstein's model, lower)

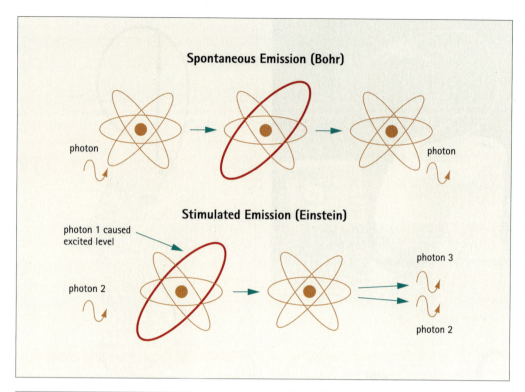

Fig. 17 Electromagnetic spectrum and dental laser wavelengths

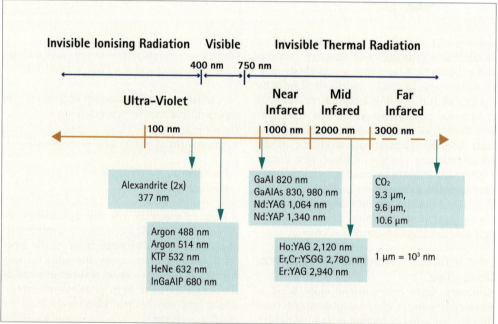

Fig. 18 Schematic of typical laser cavity. Photons are reflected back and forth, raising the energy levels of active medium atoms

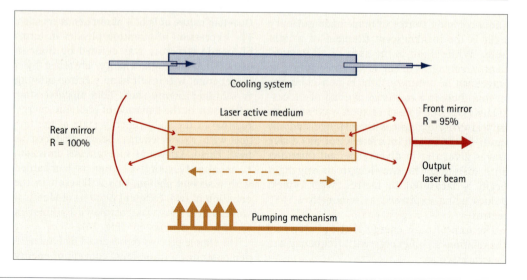

INTRODUCTION

values, ie ground state → excited state → ground state.

Laser light
Laser light occurs through the amplification of stimulated emission. Since the emission energy is unique relative to its source and of known measurable quantity, the light will be of a single wavelength (monochromatic). The high-energy, single wavelength light is produced in a spatially stable form (collimated or non-divergent), with successive waveforms that are in phase (coherent). In consequence, the coherence and collimation of the light results in high energy density and the monochromatic wavelength will define specific target absorption. These fundamental qualities will be considered in the chapter on laser-tissue interaction.

Dental laser wavelengths
With respect to the monochromatic nature of laser light, a number of emission wavelengths have been developed that, for the purposes of current clinical dentistry, span the visible to the far infrared portions of the electromagnetic spectrum (approximately 400-10,600 nm) (Fig. 17).

Components of a typical laser (Fig. 18)
The component parts of a typical laser are:

1. Active medium
A material, either naturally occurring or man-made that when stimulated, emits laser light. This material may be a solid, liquid or gas. The first 'dental' laser used a crystal of neodymium-doped yttrium aluminium garnet (Nd:YAG) as its active medium. 'YAG' is a complex crystal with the chemical composition $Y_3Al_5O_{12}$. During crystal growth, 1% neodymium (Nd^{3+}) ions are doped into the YAG crystal (Fig. 19).

Other lasers of significance in dentistry use rare earth and other metal ions within a 'doped' YAG crystal lattice, eg erbium (Er:YAG) and holmium (Ho:YAG), together with another erbium and chromium-doped garnet of yttrium, scandium and gallium (Er,Cr:YSGG).

The active medium is positioned within the laser cavity, an internally-polished tube, with mirrors co-axially positioned at each end and surrounded by the external energising input, or pumping mechanism.

The 'active medium', eg CO_2, Nd:YAG, defines the type of laser and the emission wavelength of the laser (10,600 nm and 1,064 nm respectively). Atoms of the active medium are absorbed by the process of light emission.

2. Pumping mechanism
This represents a man-made source of primary energy that excites the active medium. This is usually a light source, either a flashlight or arc-light, but can be a diode laser

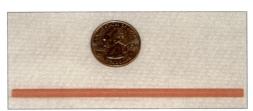

Fig. 19 A rod of Nd:YAG crystal active medium, compared to a coin to reflect the size

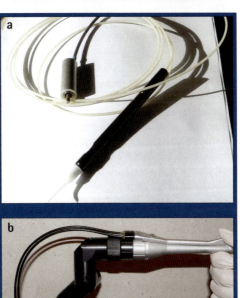

Fig. 20 A laser machine 'undressed', showing the laser cavity (active medium, optical resonator). Surrounding hardware comprises the pumping mechanism, cooling system and other circuitry

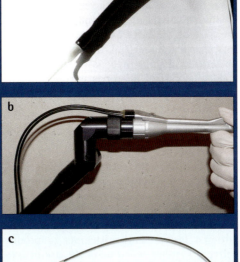
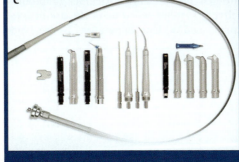
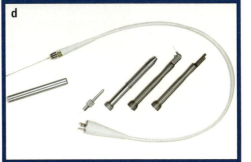

Fig. 21 Examples of different laser delivery systems, showing quartz fibre (a), articulated arm (b) and hollow waveguide (c, d)

LASERS IN DENTISTRY

Fig. 22 Example of a 'desktop' diode laser machine. Common wavelengths are KTP (532 nm), diode (810 nm) and diode (980 nm)

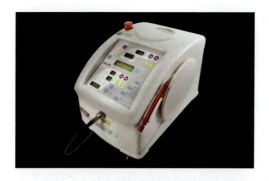

unit or an electromagnetic coil. Energy from this primary source is absorbed by the active medium, resulting in the production of laser light. This process is very inefficient, with only some 3-10% of incident energy resulting in laser light,[9] the rest being converted to heat energy.

The dynamics of incident energy with time has a fundamental bearing on the emission mode characteristics of a given laser. A continuous-feed electrical discharge will result in a similar continuous feed of laser light emission (see below, laser light emission modes).

3. Optical resonator

Laser light produced by the stimulated active medium is bounced back and forth through the axis of the laser cavity, using two mirrors placed at either end, thus amplifying the power. The distal mirror is totally reflective and the proximal mirror is partly transmissive, so that at a given energy density, laser light will escape to be transmitted to the target tissue (Fig. 20).

4. Delivery system

Dependant upon the emitted wavelength, the delivery system may be a quartz fibre-optic, a flexible hollow waveguide, an articulated arm (incorporating mirrors), or a hand-piece containing the laser unit (at present only for low-powered lasers). Early attempts to produce delivery systems relied upon the use of fixed mirror and/or lens apparatus. It was soon apparent that the use of a fine, silica quartz fibre-optic cable maximised the feasibility for medical and dental lasers to reach their target site. However, the suitability of this delivery system is conditional upon the emission wavelength being poorly absorbed by water (hydroxyl groups), present in the quartz fibre. Therefore, shorter wavelengths such as argon, diodes and Nd:YAG can enjoy such fibre delivery, whereas longer wavelengths (Er,Cr:YSGG, Er:YAG and carbon dioxide) give rise to severe power losses through quartz fibre and hence require alternative delivery systems (Fig. 21).

Examples of such alternatives are articulated arms incorporating internal mirrors and prisms, and hollow waveguides, where the light is reflected along internally-polished tubes. Newer, water-free fibre compounds, eg zirconium fluoride, are being developed to overcome this problem.[10-13]

5. Cooling system

Heat production is a by-product of laser light propagation. It increases with the power output of the laser and hence, with heavy-duty tissue cutting lasers, the cooling system represents the bulkiest component. Co-axial coolant systems may be air- or water-assisted.

6. Control panel

This allows variation in power output with time, above that defined by the pumping mechanism frequency. Other facilities may allow wavelength change (multi-laser instruments) and print-out of delivered laser energy during clinical use.

Diode lasers

The development of micro-structure diode cells that are capable of laser light production has dramatically reduced the bulk of laser machines (Fig. 22).

The limitation of the physics involved has restricted the span of spectral emissions to a relatively narrow band (approx 400-1,000 nm) at the present time. Only solid material

Fig. 23 Schematic outline of a typical diode laser. Optical reflective mirrors are replaced by polishing the respective ends of the crystals to enable internal reflection

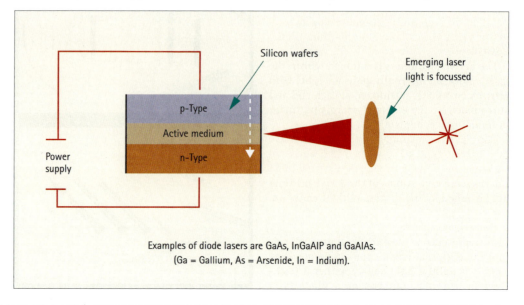

Examples of diode lasers are GaAs, InGaAlP and GaAlAs.
(Ga = Gallium, As = Arsenide, In = Indium).

INTRODUCTION

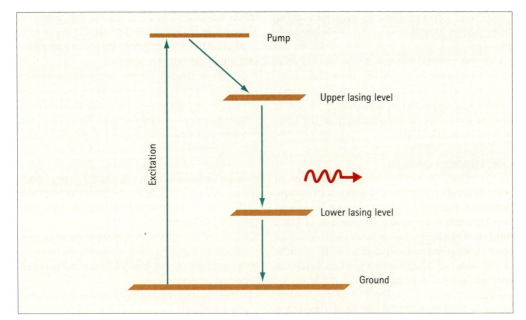

Fig. 24 Four-level energy exchange

active media are used in these lasers.

In a diode laser, the active medium is sandwiched between silicon wafers (Fig. 23). Due to the crystalline nature of the active medium, eg GaAlAs, it is possible to selectively polish the ends of the crystal relative to internal refractive indices to produce totally and partially reflective surfaces, thus replicating the optical resonators of larger lasers. The discharge of current from one silicon wafer to the other, across the active medium, releases photons from the active medium. Individual diode 'chips' produce relatively low-energy output and so current surgically-appropriate diode lasers employ banks of individual diode chips in parallel to achieve a desired power capability.

Energy exchange and wavelength emission

As was seen earlier, the ideal quantum exchange in an absorption/emission system is through a three-level transfer (ground – excited – ground). Although many lasers exhibit this (eg HeNe, N_2), several important dental laser active mediums suffer some time delay, whereby energy decay exists over a range of values, giving rise to an upper and lower lasing level of emission. This exposes the active medium to multi-wavelength emission spectra. As such, these lasers are known as four-level lasers (Fig. 24) and their relevance is such that there is a potential for a non-specific, multi-wavelength emission. However, through a choice of reflecting mirrors as optical resonators (plain, concave, convex), it is possible to create wave interference and cancellation within the laser cavity, to leave a desired emission single wavelength. This explanation accounts for the existence of, for example, a CO_2 laser at 9,300, 9,600 and 10,600 nm (Fig. 25).

The active medium of a CO_2 laser is a mixture of CO_2, helium and nitrogen gases, in proportions 8:7:1. Pumping is through an electric coil discharge. Initially, most of the electrical discharge energy is absorbed by nitrogen gas and only a small part of the energy is absorbed by CO_2 molecules directly to raise

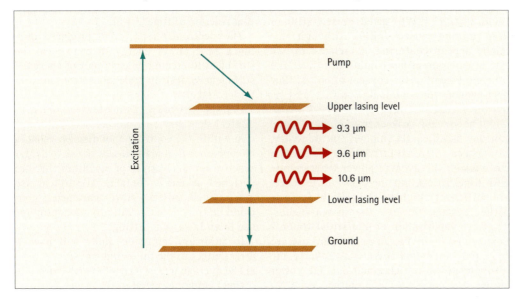

Fig. 25 CO_2 laser system

them from a ground state to the upper lasing level. Large amounts of CO_2 molecules collide with the nitrogen molecules and gain the excitation energy. Energy decay occurs over time, to a lower lasing level, thus giving out laser light at frequency 9,300 nm, 9,600 nm or 10,600 nm respectively. Remaining decay to ground state will dissipate energy in the form of heat instead of light.

Laser light beam dynamics

Collimation, one of the prime properties of laser light, is in practice a theoretical concept, in that its acceptance is based upon transmission through a vacuum. The passage of laser light through any other medium will result in some divergence with distance, which can be of the order of 15-30 degrees when using an optical fibre delivery system or a diode active medium.[14] As such, in order to be controlled, an emission beam is often passed through a focal medium, eg a bi-convex lens.

If the primary output laser beam is intersected and the transverse beam cross-section studied, the light intensity can be of different distributions (patterns), consistent with the reflective dynamics of the optical resonators. These are called transverse electromagnetic modes (TEM). Three indices are used to indicate the modes – TEM plq, where p is the number of radial zero fields, l is the number of angular zero fields and q is the number of longitudinal fields. The first two indices are usually used to specify a TEM mode, eg TEM_{00}, TEM_{10}, etc. Clearly, the higher the order of the modes the more difficult it is to focus the beam to a fine spot. TEM_{00} mode, or Gaussian beam as it is commonly known, is preferred in order to achieve desired accuracy in treatment procedures. The ability to produce a focussed beam together with the controlled application of light power over a small area, has a fundamental bearing on the concept of delivering ablation energy to a target tissue.

Laser light emission modes

Often, a clinical laser is referred to as 'continuous wave' (CW), 'gated pulsed' (GP) or 'free-running pulsed' (FRP). Although this might appear confusing, it relates to the rate of emission of laser light with time. The inherent benefit of the concept of pulsed flow over average continuous flow is that, assuming the average delivery of energy with time might be low, the peak-energy of each 'pulse' can be significantly higher. In dentistry, this is seen where an Er:YAG laser is used to cut enamel; the average power (energy rate with time) is low, but the peak power levels are sufficiently high to dislocate hydroxyapatite crystals, through the instantaneous, explosive vaporisation of interstitial water.[15] Commercial lasers for surgical dental use are commonly annotated '5 Watts', '10 Watts', etc – this relates to the maximal average power output. The emission mode epithet, eg 'CW', 'FRP' will alert the clinician to the potential peak power capacity of the laser.

In practice, the emission mode for any given laser can be either 'inherent' or 'acquired'. Inherent emission modes are related to the nature of the excitation source:
a) Free-running pulsed, where laser emission occurs over a pulse width of 100-200 microseconds
b) Continuous wave.

Acquired emission modes are due to a modifying effect (electrical, mechanical, electro-optical or acousto-optical) acting upon the inherent delivery:
a) Chopped or gated CW, where laser emission occurs over tenths (0.1-0.5) of a second
b) Q-switched, mode-locked (not applicable in dental lasers)
c) Super-pulsed, where laser emission occurs over 300-400 microseconds.

With relevance to the clinical application of any laser with any target oral tissue, it is important to consider the potential transfer of energy from the laser beam, converted to heat energy in the target, in order that only a sufficient transfer to execute designated tissue change is achieved. For a simple, low power CO_2 laser, the average power output of a CW machine is readily understood – four Watts of CW output = four Watts average power. With a FRP laser, eg Er:YAG, output is often expressed as energy per pulse and the operator can determine the number of pulses. As such, the energy per pulse, eg 200 mJ, must be multiplied by the number of pulses, eg 20 pulses per second (0.2 J x 20) to give an average power delivery of four Watts (Joules per second). The prime benefit of a pulsed delivery mode will be the capacity of the target tissue to cool between successive pulses. However, when considering a FRP laser, the peak power per pulse can be considerable. An energy-per-pulse value of 200 mJ (200 x 10^{-3} J) with a pulse duration of 100 µs (100 x 10^{-6} s) can give rise to a peak power of 2,000 Watts for that fraction of time (J ÷ s).

The electromagnetic forces produced during a peak power energy discharge can be sufficient to create a plasma ball of energy,[16] sufficient to destroy molecular structure in a target tissue.

The majority of commercial lasers for use in clinical dentistry incorporate such information within the control panel display. What is of concern is that many lasers in use in dental practice are derivatives of machines that are designed primarily for general surgical use and as such, possess power parameters that could be considered potentially damaging for use in an intra-oral setting.

In summary, emission mode will have a direct effect in the following ways:
a) The average power (rate of energy with time) being delivered to the target

INTRODUCTION

b) The peak power value of laser light being delivered to the target (observed with FRP modes)

c) The thermal relaxation effect (ability to cool) of the target.

The thermal relaxation potential is greatest in FRP emission and least in CW emission. This has a profound bearing on the tissue management during laser-tissue interaction.

1. Newton I. *Opticks: or, a treatise of the reflections, refractions, inflexions and colours of light. Also two treatises of the species and magnitude of curvilinear figures.* London, 1704.
2. Einstein A. Zur quantentheorie der strahlung. *Physiol Z* 1917; **18:** 121-128.
3. Townes C H. *Making waves.* New York: Springer-Verlag, 1994.
4. Maiman T H. Stimulated optical radiation in ruby. *Nature* 1960; **187:** 493-494.
5. Goldman L, Ingelman J M, Richfield D F. Impact of the laser on nevi and melanomas. *Arch Dermatol* 1964; **90:** 71-75.
6. Myers T D, Myers W D, Stone R M. First soft tissue study utilising a pulsed Nd YAG dental laser. *Northwest Dent* 1989; **68:** 14-17.
7. Hibst R, Keller U. Experimental studies of the application of the Er YAG laser on dental hard substances: 1. Measurement of ablation rate. *Lasers Surg Med* 1989; **9:** 338-344.
8. Bohr N. *The theory of spectra and atomic constitution.* 2nd ed. Cambridge: Cambridge University Press, 1922.
9. Prakash O, Ram R S. Simple designs to measure efficiency of different types of monochromators. *J Opt* 1996; **27:** 241-245.
10. Inberg A, Oksman M, Ben-David M, Croitoru N. Hollow waveguide for mid and thermal infrared radiation. *J Clin Laser Med Surg* 1998; **16:** 127-133.
11. Yang Y, Chaney C A, Fried N M. Erbium:YAG laser lithotripsy using hybrid germanium/silica optical fibers. *J Endourol* 2004; **18:** 830-835.
12. Konorov S O, Mitrokhin V P, Fedotov A B *et al.* Hollow-core photonic-crystal fibres for laser dentistry. *Phys Med Biol* 2004; **49:** 1359-1368.
13. Merberg G N. Current status of infrared fiber optics for medical laser power delivery. *Lasers Surg Med* 1993; **13:** 572-576.
14. Moseley H, Davison M, Allan D. Beam divergence of medical lasers. *Phys Med Biol* 1985; **30:** 853-857.
15. Apel C, Franzen R, Meister J, Sarrafzadegan H, Thelen S, Gutknecht N. Influence of the pulse duration of an Er:YAG laser system on the ablation threshold of dental enamel. *Lasers Med Sci* 2002; **17:** 253-257.
16. Hillenkamp F. Laser radiation tissue interaction. *Health Phys* 1989; **56:** 613-616.

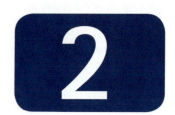

IN BRIEF

- There are two groups of lasers – 'hard', denoting surgical or cutting lasers and 'soft', denoting non-surgical, low-level devices.
- Laser light can be transmitted, reflected, scattered or absorbed by a target tissue, dependant on the absorption characteristics of the tissue.
- Laser-tissue interaction in dental surgery is primarily photothermal, in that incident energy is converted into heat. The level of heat (temperature) will define the target tissue change.
- The nature of the target tissue and a number of laser operating parameters will allow the clinician to provide precise, controlled and predictable laser-tissue interaction.

Laser-tissue interaction

The oral cavity is a unique and complex environment, where hard and soft tissues exist in close proximity, within bacteria-laden saliva. All oral tissues are receptive to laser treatment, but the biophysics governing laser-tissue interaction demands a knowledge of all factors involved in delivery of this modality; through this knowledge, correct and appropriate treatment can be delivered in a predictable manner.

LASERS IN DENTISTRY

1. Introduction, history of lasers and laser light production
2. **Laser-tissue interaction**
3. Low-level laser use in dentistry
4. Lasers and soft tissue: 'loose' soft tissue surgery
5. Lasers and soft tissue: 'fixed' soft tissue surgery
6. Lasers and soft tissue: periodontal therapy
7. Surgical laser use in implantology and endodontics
8. Surgical lasers and hard dental tissue
9. Laser regulation and safety in general dental practice

LASER TYPES USED IN TISSUE THERAPY

Anecdotally, there has evolved two groups of lasers, 'hard' and 'soft', in distinguishing their effect on tissue, although this does not relate to target tissue types. 'Hard', or surgical lasers, are essentially high power lasers which achieve desired tissue effect through a direct interaction. For the purposes of clinical dentistry, this effect is primarily photothermal[1] (Fig. 1), in that incident light energy is absorbed and converted into thermal energy which causes tissue change.

'Soft', or 'low-level' lasers are essentially low power lasers which achieve desired tissue effect through an indirect interaction, known collectively as photobiostimulation,[1] eg tissue warming, increase of local blood flow and production of 'feel-good' factors, eg endorphins. This latter group will be discussed in detail in a later chapter.

LASER-TISSUE INTERACTION

The term 'laser light' is a generic, in that one of the defining properties of laser light – that it is monochromatic – requires a qualifying emission wavelength annotation. However, the use of all laser wavelengths in clinical dentistry serves to effect controlled and precise changes in target tissue, through the transfer of electromagnetic energy.[1] A competent laser dentist will establish predictable laser-tissue interaction and all its definable outcomes, before embarking on that interaction. It is essential that through the correct choice of a given laser wavelength for treating a given target tissue, a minimum level of power is employed both to effect the desired result and to minimise the risk of collateral damage.

BASIC CONSIDERATIONS

Incident light energy will interact with a medium (eg oral tissue) that is denser than air, in one of four ways.[2] These can be listed as follows (Fig 2):

Transmission: in this way, the beam enters the medium, but there is no interaction between the incident beam and the medium. The beam will emerge distally, unchanged or partially refracted.

Scatter: there is some interaction, but this is insufficient to cause complete attenuation of the beam. Scatter will cause some diminution of light energy with distance, together with a distortion in the beam, whereby rays proceed in an uncontrolled direction through the medium. Back-scatter of the laser beam can occur as it hits the tissue; this is seen most in short wavelengths, eg diode, Nd:YAG (≥50% back-scatter).

Reflection: the density of the medium, or angle of incidence being less than the refractive angle, results in a total reflection of the beam. In true reflection, the incident and

TISSUE INTERACTION

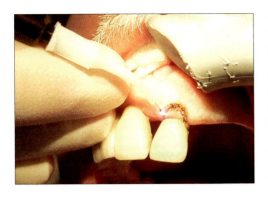

emergence angles will be the same or, if the medium interface is rough or non-homogenous, some scatter may occur.

Absorption: the incident energy of the beam is attenuated by the medium and transferred into another form. In clinical dentistry, depending on the value of the energy, there will be a conversion into heat or, in the case of very low values, biostimulation of receptor tissue sites. This can be readily appreciated through an analogy of sun-bathing – the stimulation of 'tanning' melanocytes by low-grade UV sunlight *versus* the damaging sun-burn with higher exposure values.

In any desired laser-tissue interaction, the achievement of maximum absorption by the target tissue of the incident laser energy will allow a maximal control of the resultant effects, summarised as follows:

- Absorption is determined by matching incident energy (wavelength) to the electron shell energy in target atoms.

Fig. 1 The use of a diode (810 nm) laser in this crown lengthening procedure illustrates the 'photothermal' nature of laser-tissue interaction. Incident electromagnetic (light) energy is absorbed by gingival pigmented tissue and converted to heat, which effects tissue ablation

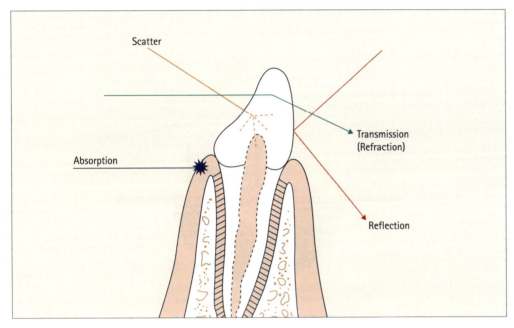

Fig. 2 Incident laser light interaction with tissue – event possibilities

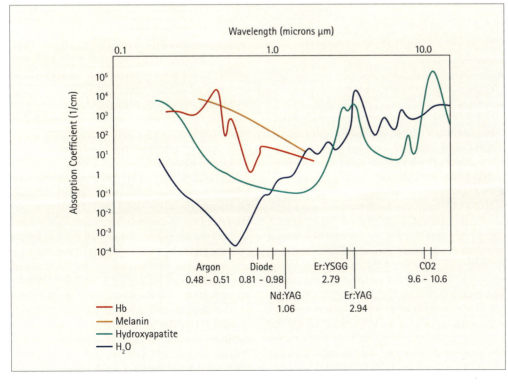

Fig. 3 Outline absorption coefficients (haemoglobin, melanin, hydroxyapatite and water) relative to laser wavelength

Fig. 4 Power density effects due to the change in spot size of a focused laser beam. This effect relates to the contact (or non-contact) of the laser hand-piece with the target tissue

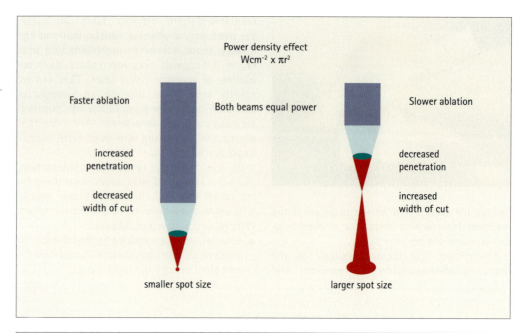

Fig. 5 Theoretical zones of tissue change associated with soft tissue exposure to laser light

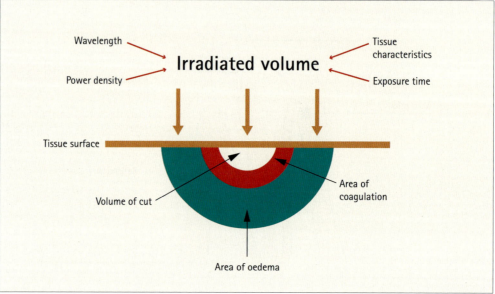

In addition, with regard to surgical laser-tissue interaction:
- Absorption of incident energy leads to generation of heat
- Ascending heat levels leads to dissociation of covalent bonds (in tissue proteins), phase transfer from liquid to vapour (in intra- and inter-cellular water), onto phase transfer to hydrocarbon gases and production of residual carbon[3]
- Heat generation can lead to secondary effects through conduction.

The physical change in target tissue achieved through heat transfer is termed photothermolysis. This is further sub-divided, subject to temperature change, phase transfer and incident energy levels, into photopyrolysis, photovaporolysis and photoplasmolysis:

Photopyrolysis: consistent with ascending temperature change from 60°C to 90°C, target tissue proteins undergo morphologic change, which is predominately permanent.

Photovaporolysis: at 100°C, inter- and intra-cellular water in soft tissue and interstitial water in hard tissue is vaporised. This destructive phase transfer results in expansive volume change, which can aid the ablative effect of the laser by dissociating large tissue elements, especially seen in laser use in hard dental tissue cutting.

Photoplasmolysis: characterised by high temperatures and explosive expansion at micro-tissue and molecular levels, this is observed in ultra-short pulsed lasers, eg Nd:YAG, Er:YAG, with pulse widths of <100 µs. This phenomenon is adjunctive to photothermolysis, whereby a plasma is formed by the ionising effects of the strong electric fields of light waves, and power densities $>10^{10}$ W/cm^2 are attained.[4] Photoplasmolysis is achieved photonically in soft tissue and thermionically in hard tissue and is characterised by flashes and popping sounds during laser use. Plasma formation can be beneficial, in that extremely high ablative energies can be produced, but

TISSUE INTERACTION

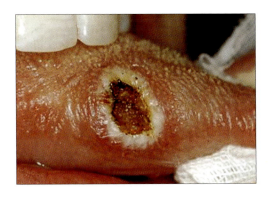

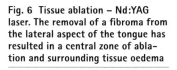

Fig. 6 Tissue ablation – Nd:YAG laser. The removal of a fibroma from the lateral aspect of the tongue has resulted in a central zone of ablation and surrounding tissue oedema

also disruptive in that it can 'shield' the target from further incident light, through the phenomenon of a plasma acting as a 'super-absorber' of electromagnetic radiation. It is considered that, within therapeutic levels of laser power used in dental procedures, photoplasmolysis is a rare occurrence.

THERMAL RELAXATION

The conversion of electromagnetic energy to heat effects in target tissue can only be deemed predictable if unwanted change through conductive thermal spread is prevented. Thermal relaxation is the term applied to the ability to control a progressively increasing heat loading of target tissue.[5] Assuming fixed values of thermal and light diffusivity for any given tissue, thermal relaxation rates are proportional to the area of tissue exposed and inversely proportional to the absorption coefficient of the tissue. Factors that influence thermal relaxation can be listed as follows.

Laser absorption characteristics

Laser emission mode, duty cycle: laser light can be emitted as a continuous beam, or in varying forms of pulses with time. Any pulsing of laser light delivery will allow some cooling to occur. Thermal relaxation will occur least with continuous wave emission and maximally in free-running pulsed delivery, with frequent operator-chosen time intervals.

Laser incident power (Joules per second)

Laser power density (Watts per square centimetre): for any chosen level of incident power, the smaller the beam diameter, the greater concentration of heat effects.

Beam movement: relative to tissue site; rapid laser beam movement will reduce heat build-up and aid thermal relaxation.

Endogenous coolant: blood flow.

Exogenous coolant: water, air, pre-cooling of tissue.[6,7]

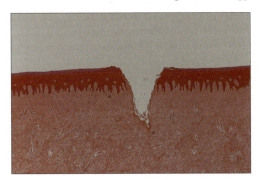

Fig. 7 CO_2 laser and oral epithelium. The zone of ablation is characteristically 'V' shaped, reflecting little conductive heat effects

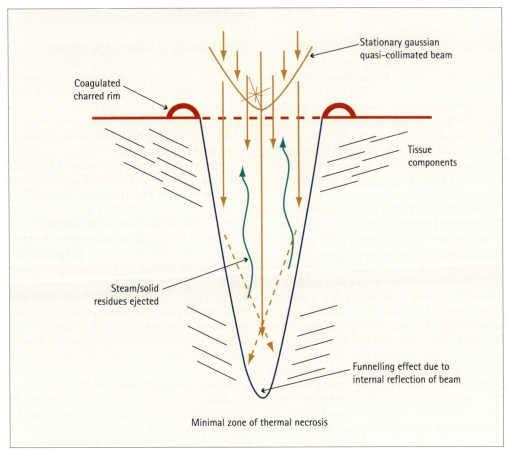

Fig. 8 CO_2 laser interaction with soft tissue. This schematic illustration identifies the vaporisation and dispersal of water within the target tissue

LASERS IN DENTISTRY

Fig. 9 Diode laser and oral epithelium. Due to deeper penetration and conductive heat effects, the zone of ablation is more rounded in outline

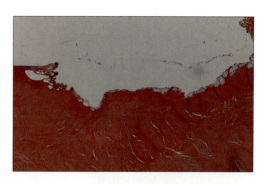

SECONDARY FACTORS AFFECTING ABSORPTION

The following factors will each and collectively affect the absorption of laser light by a target tissue:[8]

- Laser wavelength
- Tissue (composition)
- Tissue thickness
- Surface wetness
- Incident angle of beam
- Exposure time
- Contact *vs* non-contact modes.

Fig. 10 Diode laser cutting and soft tissue schematic

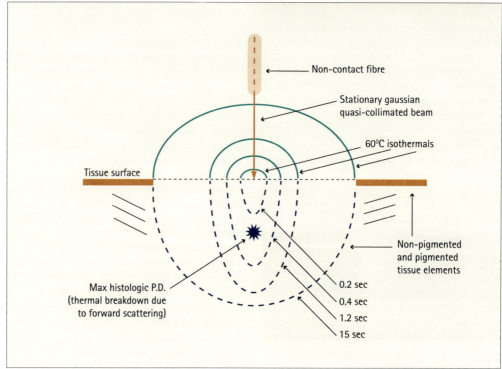

Laser wavelength and tissue composition

Tissue elements that absorb laser light energy are termed chromophores. Oral tissue can be considered as composed of one or more chromophores – haemoglobin, melanin and allied pigmented proteins, (carbonated) hydroxyapatite, and water. Relative to the spectrum of laser wavelengths currently in use in clinical dentistry, the absorption coefficients of these chromophores are shown in Figure 3.

In using the minimum amount of incident energy to effect a desired tissue change, it can be summarised that, with regard to current use of lasers in clinical practice, any tissue that is predominately pigmented will absorb shorter, ie visible and near infra-red, laser wavelengths, whereas non-pigmented tissue will absorb longer wavelengths. In addition, absorption peaks of water and (carbonated) hydroxyapatite, coincident with Er:YAG, Er:YSGG and CO_2 wavelengths, would support the potentially advantageous use of these lasers in hard tissue management. However, the prime interaction based on absorption peaks is often compromised by other factors, as discussed below.

Tissue thickness and depth of penetration

The existence of water as a constituent of all living tissue will influence the penetration of longer wavelength laser light, whilst non-pigmented surface components will prove transmissive to shorter wavelengths, leading to potentially deep penetration. In this way, whereas CO_2 wavelength might penetrate oral epithelium to a depth of 0.1-0.2 mm, Nd:YAG and diode wavelengths can result in an equivalent-power penetration of 4-6 mm.[9]

Incident angle of beam and surface wetting

The control of laser-tissue interaction is maximised if the incident beam is perpendicular to the tissue surface. As the incident angle reduces towards the refractive angle of the tissue surface, so the potential for true light reflection becomes more apparent, with an associated reduction in tissue change.[10] Surface wetness is less of a problem for shorter wavelength use.

Emission mode and exposure time

As discussed earlier, the emission mode will affect the potential for any peak energy values; equally the thermal relaxation benefits, both inherent with low duty cycle

TISSUE INTERACTION

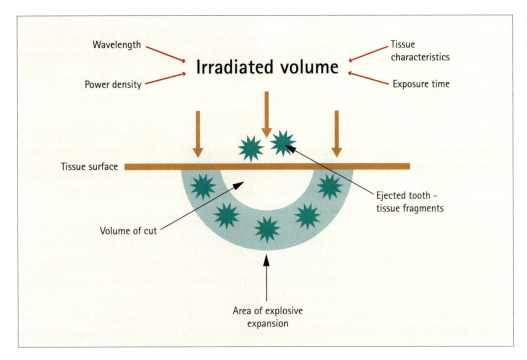

Fig. 11 Theoretical zone of tissue change associated with hard dental tissue exposure to laser light

emissions and applied through power-off intervals, will enhance therapeutic tissue management.

Contact *vs* non-contact modes
Laser light will undergo some divergence on exit from a quartz fibre delivery system and most non-fibre systems (hollow waveguide and articulated arm) use a focusing lens. Consequently, the 'spot size' of the beam, relative to the target tissue, will determine the concentration of laser energy – fluence and power density – being delivered over an area.[11] The spot size will change with distance for any delivery system – it will increase with distance for a fibre-optic delivered beam and change relative to the focal length of the lens in those delivery systems where a focusing hand-piece is used (Fig. 4).

It follows, therefore, that during any laser-tissue interaction the concentration of energy being delivered to a target site can be modified and controlled by moving the hand-piece back and forth. In this way, thermal changes can be effectively controlled.

LASER LIGHT AND SOFT TISSUE
Figures 5 and 6 depict a schematic and clinical example of an ideal surgical laser interaction with soft tissue. Assuming a correct

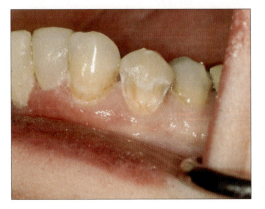

Fig. 12 Class V cavity preparation carried out using an Er:YAG laser

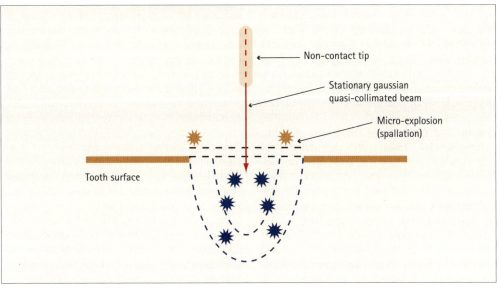

Fig. 13 Schematic progressive micro-explosion ablation of dental hard tissue with mid-infrared (Er:YAG, Er,Cr:YSGG) laser wavelengths

LASERS IN DENTISTRY

Fig. 14 Scanning electron micrographs showing the effects of Er:YAG laser light on enamel. Note the fragmentation of tissue edges and lack of conductive thermal effects

Fig. 15 Scanning electron micrograph showing the cutting effect of Er:YAG laser light on bone

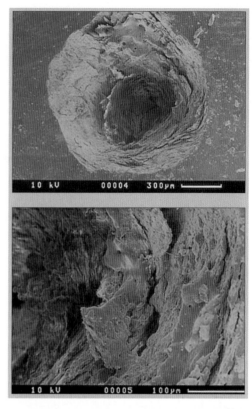

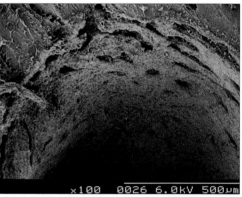

incident wavelength, using correct delivery parameters, a central zone of tissue ablation is surrounded by an area of irreversible protein denaturation (coagulation, eschar). Surrounding this, along a thermal gradient, a reversible, reactionary zone of oedema will develop. The depth and extent of this tissue change will differ with laser wavelength, being more superficial in nature with longer wavelengths, with less oedema, and deeper with greater oedema with shorter wavelengths.

Soft tissue cutting dynamics and laser wavelength

A distinct difference can be observed between short and long laser wavelengths, in their interaction with soft tissue. Longer wavelengths, being maximally absorbed by water-based chromophores, exhibit a sharp surface-configured interaction, with little sub-surface disruption[12] (Figs 7 and 8).

Shorter wavelengths give rise to a greater zone of deeper disruption, accentuated through conductive heat transfer (Figs 9 and 10).

Generally, with laser use on soft tissue, there is minimal or no bleeding. This is due to a combination of small vessels being sealed through tissue protein denaturation and stimulation of Factor VII production in clotting. The incision line will at best equal the beam diameter, and the production of a surface coagulum obviates need for sutures. Healing will always be by secondary intention and little or no scar formation is seen to occur. Compared to scalpel incisions, the healing time is delayed, although, due to the coagulum layer, there is little potential for bacterial contamination of the wound.[13]

LASER USE AND HARD TISSUE

Figures 11 and 12 illustrate the theoretical and clinical effects of long wavelength laser light on hard dental tissue. Potentially, unlike laser wavelengths and soft tissue chromophores, there are three wavelengths that will interact with dental hard tissue. The predominant two are Er:YAG (2,940 nm) and Er,Cr:YSGG (2,780 nm),[14] together with CO_2 (10,600 nm). These wavelengths have an affinity for (carbonated) hydroxyapatite and water chromophores. However, although the water content of enamel and dentine is very low (3-5% in enamel and 13-15% in dentine), it is the configuration of the emission modes in commercial dental lasers that defines the underlying nature of tissue ablation. The commonly-employed wavelength of CO_2 lasers in dentistry (10,600 nm) has a high absorption in water, but a relatively low absorbance in hydroxyapatite when compared to the 9,600 nm wavelength found in laboratory CO_2 lasers. In addition, the 10,600 nm CO_2 laser emits in continuous and gated-continuous wave modes, which not only renders the average power output low, but also significantly reduces the thermal relaxation potential. This can have disastrous effects with dental hard tissues.[15]

Equally, the use of shorter wavelengths, eg Nd:YAG (1,064 nm), which have no appreciable absorption in dental hard tissue, can lead to thermal cracking and amorphous change in the hydroxyapatite crystal structure. In addition, there is a potential for high intra-pulpal temperature rise, due to transmission of this laser energy through enamel and dentine.[16]

Hard tissue cutting dynamics and laser wavelength

Both erbium laser wavelengths have free-running pulsed emission modes, which give rise to high peak power levels (>1,000 Watts). Such power levels result in an instantaneous, explosive vaporisation of the water content of enamel and dentine, which leads to dissociation of the tissue and ejection of microfragments (Figs 13 and 14). In addition, both

TISSUE INTERACTION

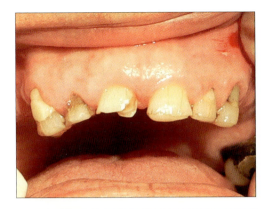

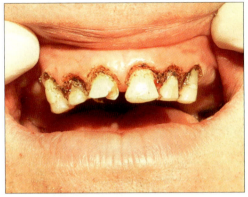

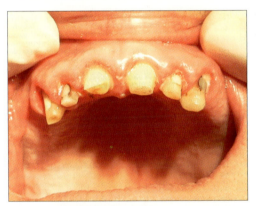

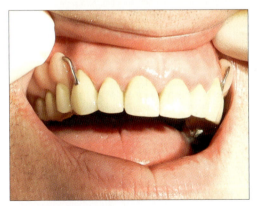

lasers use co-axial water spray to aid dispersal of ablated tissue and to cool the target.[17] In comparison with rotary instrumentation, pulpal temperature rise is minimal when erbium laser wavelengths are employed.[18] As such, cavity preparation proceeds without surface cracking.

It has been shown that the crater depth and ablation volume during enamel and dentine ablation proceed in a linear relationship with time. However, if the auxiliary water spray is prevented from reaching the cavity, the build-up of ablation debris prevents further cutting and there is consequent heat production.

Laser ablation of bone with erbium laser wavelengths proceeds in a similar fashion. The higher water content and lower density of bone compared to enamel allows faster cutting, through dislocation of hydroxyapatite and cleavage of the collagen matrix (Fig. 15).

This ease of cutting places the use of Er:YAG and Er,Cr:YSGG laser wavelengths as the preferred choice for laser bone ablation when compared to other wavelengths, although there may be slightly higher heating effects with Er:YSGG.[19]

The use of erbium YAG and YSGG laser wavelengths in the ablation and management of root dentine and cementum results in efficient and clean removal of tissue, due to the relatively high water content. The correct use of laser power parameters, together with adequate water spray, prevents direct thermal damage to the tissue structure, witnessed by the absence of melting or cracking.[20] As with other dental hard tissue, the use of CO_2 laser, in its dentally configured form, should be avoided.[21]

BENEFITS OF LASER–TISSUE INTERACTION
From the above, a number of benefits of laser use in the treatment of soft and hard tissue can be listed as follows:

Soft tissue:
- Ability to cut, coagulate, ablate or vaporise target tissue elements
- Sealing of small blood vessels (dry field of surgery)
- Sealing of small lymphatic vessels (reduced post-operative oedema)
- Sterilising of tissue (due to heat build-up and production of eschar layer and destruction of bacterial forms)
- Decreased post-operative tissue shrinkage (decreased amount of scarring).

Hard tissue:
- Ability to selectively ablate carious dental tissue (faster ablation due to higher water content)
- Reduced peri-operative cracking compared to rotary instrumentation
- Scope for minimally-invasive restorative treatment of early caries
- Reduced pulpal temperature rise
- Cavity sterilisation.

Examples of the advantages of laser-tissue interaction in delivering general dental treatment are given in Figures 16-23. The ability to ablate diseased or excess tissue elements whilst minimising unwanted extraneous effects, and to combine otherwise-staged treatment, defines real benefit to both the clinician and the patient.

Fig. 16 Pre-operative combined crown lengthening, fixed and removable prosthetics case

Fig. 17 Use of CO_2 laser to remove excess gingival tissue and re-contour soft tissue profile

Fig. 18 Healing soft tissue at two weeks

Fig. 19 Completed treatment at six weeks

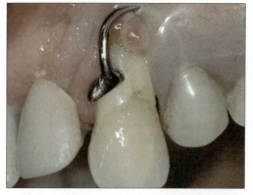
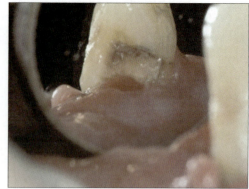
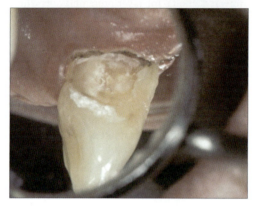
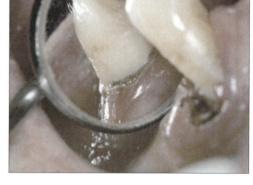

Fig. 20 (left) Denture-induced epulis and class V cavity at UL canine

Fig. 21 (right) Partial denture removed to show hard and soft tissue lesions

Fig. 22 (left) Hyperaemic epulis removed using diode laser to induce haemostasis, cervical margin of cavity exposed using CO_2 laser and cavity preparation completed using Er:YAG laser

Fig. 23 (right) Completed single-visit treatment

1. Knappe V, Frank F, Rohde E. Principles of lasers and biophotonic effects. *Photomed Laser Surg* 2004; **22:** 411-417.
2. Ball K A. *Lasers: the perioperative challenge.* 2nd ed. pp 14-17. St Louis: Mosby-Year Book, 1995.
3. Moshonov J, Stabholz A, Leopold Y, Rosenberg I, Stabholz A. Lasers in dentistry. Part B – interaction with biological tissues and the effect on the soft tissues of the oral cavity, the hard tissues of the tooth and the dental pulp. *Refuat Hapeh Vehashinayim* 2001; **18:** 21-28, 107-108.
4. Hillenkamp F. Laser radiation tissue interaction. *Health Phys* 1989; **56:** 613-616.
5. van Gemert M J, Lucassen G W, Welch A J. Time constants in thermal laser medicine: II. Distributions of time constants and thermal relaxation of tissue. *Phys Med Biol* 1996; **41:** 1381-1399.
6. Anvari B, Motamedi M, Torres J H, Rastegar S, Orihuela E. Effects of surface irrigation on the thermal response of tissue during laser irradiation. *Lasers Surg Med* 1994; **14:** 386-395.
7. Pinheiro A L, Browne R M, Frame J W, Matthews J B. Mast cells in laser and surgical wounds. *Braz Dent J* 1995; **6:** 11-15.
8. Dederich D N. Laser/tissue interaction: what happens to laser light when it strikes tissue? *J Am Dent Assoc* 1993; **124:** 57-61.
9. Ball K A. *Lasers: the perioperative challenge.* 2nd ed. pp 19. St Louis: Mosby-Year Book, 1995.
10. Gaspar L, Kasler M, Orosz M. Effect of CO_2 laser beam angle of incidence in the oral cavity. *J Clin Laser Med Surg* 1991; **9:** 209-213.
11. Myers T D, Murphy D G, White J M, Gold S I. Conservative soft tissue management with the low-powered pulsed Nd:YAG dental laser. *Pract Periodont Aesthet Dent* 1992; **4:** 6-12.
12. Fisher J C. Photons, physiatrics, and physicians: a practical guide to understanding laser light interaction with living tissue, part I. *J Clin Laser Med Surg* 1992; **10:** 419-426.
13. Fisher S E, Frame J W, Browne R M, Tranter R M. A comparative histological study of wound healing following CO_2 laser and conventional surgical excision of canine buccal mucosa. *Arch Oral Biol* 1983; **28:** 287-291.
14. Wigdor H, Abt E, Ashrafi S, Walsh JT Jr. The effect of lasers on dental hard tissues. *J Am Dent Assoc* 1993; **124:** 65-70.
15. Launay Y, Mordon S, Cornil A, Brunetaud J M, Moschetto Y. Thermal effects of lasers on dental tissues. *Lasers Surg Med* 1987; **7:** 473-477.
16. Allen D J. Thermal effects associated with the Nd/YAG dental laser. *Angle Orthod* 1993; **63:** 299-303.
17. Hoke J A, Burkes E J Jr, Gomes E D, Wolbarsht M L. Erbium: YAG (2.94 mum) laser effects on dental tissues. *J Laser Appl* 1990; **2:** 61-65.
18. Rizoiu I, Kohanghadosh F, Kimmel A I, Eversole L R. Pulpal thermal responses to an erbium,chromium:YSGG pulsed laser hydrokinetic system. *Oral Surg Oral Med Oral Pathol Oral Radiol Endod* 1998; **86:** 220-223.
19. Jahn R, Bleckmann A, Duczynski E *et al.* Thermal side effects after use of the pulsed IR laser on meniscus and bone tissue. *Unfallchirurgie* 1994; **20:** 1-10.
20. Sasaki K M, Aoki A, Ichinose S, Ishikawa I. Morphological analysis of cementum and root dentin after Er:YAG laser irradiation. *Lasers Surg Med* 2002; **31:** 79-85.
21. Anic I, Dzubur A, Vidovic D, Tudja M. Temperature and surface changes of dentine and cementum induced by CO_2 laser exposure. *Int Endod J* 1993; **26:** 284-293.

IN BRIEF

- Low-level, non-cutting lasers are commonly used in many areas of general medicine and veterinary practice.
- Their use in treating pathology is based on photobiostimulation, in which laser energy is absorbed by inter- and intra-cellular targets, resulting in a secondary stimulation of tissue healing mechanisms.
- In dentistry, a number of clinical conditions affecting the teeth and jaws may be amenable to low-level laser therapy.
- Photo-dynamic therapy, where a drug or chemical is introduced and activated by laser light, can be used in dentistry to treat bacterial infection in endodontics and periodontology.
- Additional uses of low-level laser light include caries detection and scanning techniques in orthodontics and restorative dentistry.

Low-level laser use in dentistry

The use of laser light at power levels below that capable of direct tissue change (protein denaturation, water vaporisation and tissue ablation), has been advocated in diverse branches of medicine and veterinary practice, yet its acceptance in general dental practice remains low. However, the scope for using low-level laser light (LLLT) has emerged through many applications, either directly or indirectly tissue-related, in delivering primary dental care. The purpose of this chapter is to explain the mechanisms of action and to explore the uses of this group of lasers in general dental practice.

LASERS IN DENTISTRY

1. Introduction, history of lasers and laser light production
2. Laser-tissue interaction
3. **Low-level laser use in dentistry**
4. Lasers and soft tissue: 'loose' soft tissue surgery
5. Lasers and soft tissue: 'fixed' soft tissue surgery
6. Lasers and soft tissue: periodontal therapy
7. Surgical laser use in implantology and endodontics
8. Surgical lasers and hard dental tissue
9. Laser regulation and safety in general dental practice

THE USES OF LOW-LEVEL LASERS IN GENERAL DENTAL PRACTICE

A number of applications of low-level laser light have emerged, which utilise either the specific wavelength/chromophore relationship, or the inherent accuracy of a collimated beam. The most significant uses are listed as follows:

- Photobiostimulation
- Composite resin curing
- Caries detection
- Photo-activated disinfection (PAD)
- Laser scanning (restorative dentistry, orthodontics)

PHOTOBIOSTIMULATION
Background
The therapeutic effects of sunlight in treating a wide range of diseases has been recognised over many centuries, and are known collectively as heliotherapy. Systemic diseases, ranging from dementia and tuberculosis to skin diseases such as lupus vulgaris and acne, were commonly treated in the early part of the 20th century by exposure to sun and other natural light. The development of treatments involving UV light, actinotherapy and photomedicine led to positive effects in helping patients suffering from rickets (vitamin D deficiency), together with claims of healing boils, carbuncles, neo-natal jaundice and for pain relief.[1-3]

Following the production of the first laser in 1960, itself a comparatively low-powered instrument, research into other lasers such as helium-neon (633 nm) followed. In Eastern Europe in the late 1960s, workers such as Mester,[4] encouraged by laboratory experiments into regenerative healing effects in mice, treated patients with open wounds where conventional therapies had failed, reporting success rates of 85%. During the 1970s and 1980s, the popularity of LLLT therapies grew, mainly in Europe and Asia, and with it, the development of diode lasers (GaAS 904 nm, GaAlAs 780-890 nm and, latterly, InGaAlP 630-700 nm). All these lasers have deep penetrating potential in tissue and are portable, easy to use and relatively inexpensive. The use of these wavelengths centred around research that supported claims of benefits in treating musculo-skeletal, neuro-muscular, cytogenic and trauma-related conditions through biologic effects known as photobiostimulation. The underlying principle is that improvement in a condition is through stimulation of cellular and biochemically-mediated (essentially indirect) elements.[5]

Application of LLLT in photobiostimulation
The triage of dental treatment can be summarised as the control/eradication of disease, the control/relief of pain, and the restoration of form/function. The inter-relationship of

LASERS IN DENTISTRY

Fig. 1 'The circle of suffering' inter-relationship between stimulus, response and pain

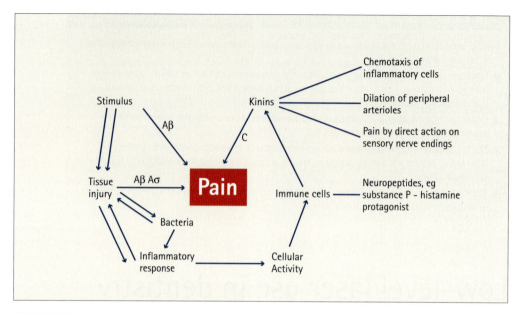

Fig. 2 Self-contained low level laser device (figure courtesy of Dr G. Ross, Toronto)

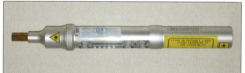

any stimulus with injury, cellular response and pain can be the product of the nature and potency of the stimulus and the ability of the tissue to respond (Fig. 1). Research on peri-apical lesions has shown that there is a correlation between the release of cellular and biochemical mediators and the nature of the injury, with acute and traumatic injuries resulting in greater reactive processes, compared to chronic pathogenesis.[6]

Low-level laser therapy (photobiostimulation) involves the use of visible red and near-infrared light with tissue in order to stimulate and improve healing, as well as reduce pain. The incident wavelength determines the effect – visible light is transmitted through the superficial cellular layers (eg the dermis, epidermis and the subcutaneous tissue). Light waves in the near-infrared ranges potentially penetrate several millimetres and these wavelengths are used to stimulate deep cellular function. Light energy is absorbed within living tissue by cellular photoreceptors, eg cytochromophores. The incident electromagnetic energy is converted by cellular mitochondria into ATP (adenosine tri-phosphate), a product of cytochrome c-oxidase activity and the Krebs cycle.[7] Consequently, the stimulated increase in ATP production would suggest an increased cellular activity in eg fibroblasts, involved in tissue healing.[8] In addition, the conversion of some of the incident energy into heat would suggest an increase in local micro-circulation through vasodilation.

The stimulatory effects of LLLT include the following:[9-13]

- Proliferation of macrophages
- Proliferation of lymphocytes
- Proliferation of fibroblasts
- Proliferation of endothelial cells
- Proliferation of keratinocytes
- Increased cell respiration/ATP synthesis
- Release of growth factors and other cytokines
- Transformation of fibroblasts into myofibroblasts
- Collagen synthesis.

In addition, there is evidence to support the analgesic effects of LLLT, through an enhanced synthesis of endorphins and bradykinins, decreased c-fibre activity and altered pain threshold.[14,15] Other research suggests a therapeutic analgesic effect, through the release of serotonin and acetylcholine centrally, and histamine and prostaglandins peripherally, with the use of LLLT.[16]

Laser units

In comparison to surgical lasers, low-level laser units are much smaller, often self-contained, hand-held devices (Fig. 2), which are either battery-driven or charged via a pod in a bench-top master unit. There is no need for any integral cooling system and their power output levels often warrant no specific safety rules that apply to surgical laser units.

The dosimetry of low-level laser light is crucial to the infra-surgical effects of the wavelengths used. This is based on the Arndt Schultz law,[17] summarised as 'small doses stimulate living systems, medium doses impede, and large doses destroy'. This is illustrated in a study carried out where hamster ovarian cells were exposed to varying low laser energy.[18] The incident fluence, increasing through a range of infra-ablative values, gave rise to cellular effects as follows:

a) <60 mJ/cm^2 – zero bio-activation
b) 120-240 mJ/cm^2 – bio-stimulation
c) 240-300 mJ/cm^2 – zero bio-activation
d) 300-600 mJ/cm^2 – bio-inhibition (release of cellular singlet oxygen).

LOW-LEVEL LASERS

The amount of laser energy delivered to a target tissue is termed fluence, or energy density and is measured in J/cm^2. The power of the laser light is the product of fluence and time, which for a free-running emission mode can result in peak power values of several thousand Watts, albeit for periods of micro-seconds. With surgical or cutting lasers, vaporisation of intra- and inter-cellular water occurs at fluence levels of 1,000 J/cm^2.[19] In clinical practice, low-level laser therapy, effective through stimulatory rather than ablative mechanisms, delivers fluence of 2-10 J/cm^2, depending on the target tissue[20] as follows:

- Oral epithelium and gingival tissue – 2-3 J/cm^2
- Trans-osseous irradiation (target – peri-apical area) – 2-4 J/cm^2
- Extra-oral muscle groups/TMJ – 6-10 J/cm^2.

Clinical applications in dental practice

It is perhaps best to consider the scope of application of LLLT in dentistry through the underlying cellular mechanism, rather than the descriptive clinical term. For example, tooth hypersensitivity may be viewed as an inflammatory condition and an extraction socket as post-trauma. In this way, the use of LLLT is to stimulate the inherent cellular and biochemical pathways associated with resolution and healing (Figs 3-5).

Reported effects in clinical dentistry include the following:

- Dentine hypersensitivity[21]
- Post-extraction socket/post-trauma sites[22]
- Viral infections: herpes labialis, herpes simplex[23,24]
- Neuropathy: trigeminal neuralgia, paraesthesia[25]
- Apthous ulceration[26]
- TMJDS[25]
- Post-oncology: mucositis, dermatitis, post-surgery healing.[27]

LLLT – the debate?

Despite the numbers of published studies (2,500+), of which more than 100 are positive and double-blind, the acceptance of low-level lasers in primary dental therapy remains guarded. Approval and scepticism are curiously divided by geographical location, with greatest acceptance being expressed in Northern and Eastern Europe and Asia. Claims to the magnitude of the placebo effect in studies continue to fuel the lack of objective analysis.[28] There is an increasing popularity being expressed in North America for LLLT use in dental practice and, whilst clinicians may choose to include such modalities in their practice, the need for wider-ranging evidence-based research must remain paramount, both for the credibility of this treatment and with respect to patients.

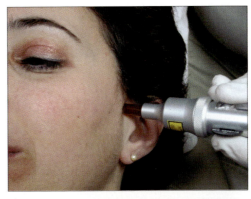

Fig. 3 TMJ stimulation (figure courtesy of Dr G. Ross, Toronto)

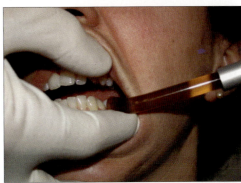

Fig. 4 Tooth hypersensitivity (figure courtesy of Dr G. Ross, Toronto)

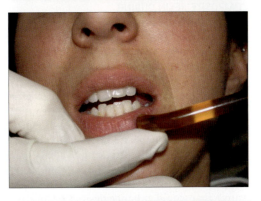

Fig. 5 Herpes labialis (figure courtesy of Dr G. Ross, Toronto)

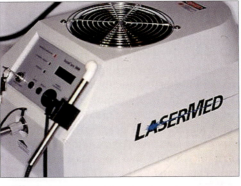

Fig. 6 Argon curing laser (LaserMed UK)

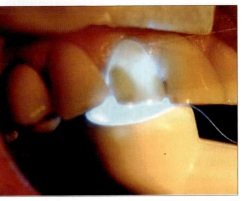

Fig. 7 Argon curing light

Fig. 8 (left) DiagnoDENT (Kavo GmbH)

Fig. 9 (right) Laser probe in use

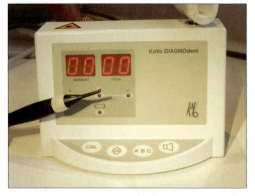
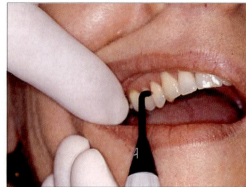

Fig. 10 (left) Occlusal scan

Fig. 11 (right) Interstitial scan

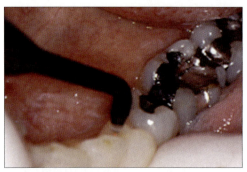
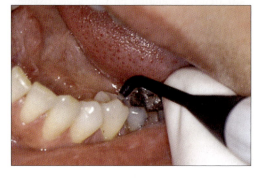

COMPOSITE RESIN CURING

One of the major emission wavelengths of argon lasers is the 488 nm 'blue'. This wavelength coincides with the absorption peak of camphorquinone, an accelerator used in composite resin restorative materials. The early work carried out on the effectiveness of a high density prime wavelength light source, suggested that the depth of curing and hardness of the set composite offered advantages over contemporary light curing systems.[29-32] The intensity of the incident laser beam, using low power levels (150-300 mW) offered a light source that would enhance desired restorative properties without excessive pulpal temperature rise.

Unfortunately, the duality of emission wavelengths of the argon active medium required selective filtering of the longer, 514 nm 'green' (soft tissue ablative) wavelength, together with the limitation of the hardware required to restrict emission light energy. Consequently, argon laser curing units were expensive and rendered suitable only for composite curing and some laser whitening uses (Figs 6 and 7). In addition, the simultaneous development of more powerful curing systems (eg plasma-arc curing lights), offered similar results without the cost and peripheral safety requirements of the laser unit.

CARIES DETECTION

Although the use of fluorescence had been suggested for caries detection already more than a century ago, the current optical caries detection techniques emerged with the introduction of laser technology into the dental field. In the 1980s, a clinically applicable visual detection[33,34] method focussing on the natural green fluorescence of tooth tissue was developed. The technique used a 488 nm excitation wavelength from an argon-ion laser to discriminate bright green fluorescing healthy tooth tissue from poorly fluorescing caries lesions. The technique was developed further in the early 1990s, into what is now known as quantitative light-induced fluorescence (QLF),[35,36] using the digitisation of fluorescence images to quantify the observed green fluorescence loss as an indirect measure of mineral loss.

Around that time, in veterinary dental research and human dental research, a red fluorescence method emerged. The red fluorescence, excited either using long UV (350-410 nm) or red (550-670 nm) wavelengths, was observed in advanced caries as well as plaque and calculus on teeth.[37,38] Opposite to the green fluorescence loss observed in caries, a substantial red fluorescence occurs between 650 and 800 nm in caries lesions that is much brighter than that of sound enamel or dentine.[39-41]

The first commercially available unit using a red laser was manufactured by Kavo (Kavo GmbH) in 1998, with an emission wavelength of 655 nm (Fig. 8). The effectiveness of this system is deemed to be best incorporated as an adjunct to other diagnostic methods (tactile, visual, radiographic), to limit the possibility of 'false positive' results, which is borne out in recent studies.[42] Nonetheless, the unit, which offers a reproducible analogue scoring of site examination, allows a degree of objective assay of those suspect areas of caries that are subject to on-going review as to treatment. Primarily, the use of this modality has been to detect occlusal or flat surface defects, although interstitial caries can be recorded (Figs 9-11). The presence of existing

LOW-LEVEL LASERS

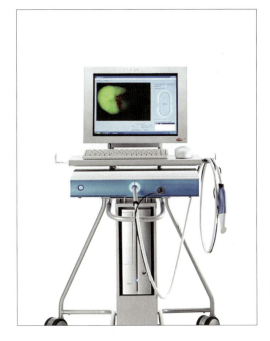

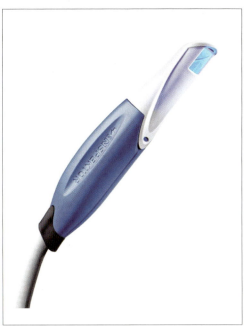

Fig. 12 (left) Quantitative light-induced fluorescence. QLF unit and computer hardware (courtesy of Inspektor Dental Care BV, Amsterdam, NL)

Fig. 13 (right) QLF hand-piece (courtesy of Inspektor Dental Care BV, Amsterdam, NL)

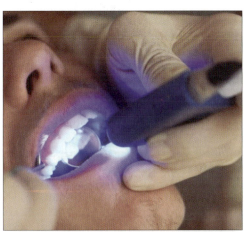

Fig. 14 QLF unit in use in the mouth (courtesy of Inspektor Dental Care BV, Amsterdam, NL)

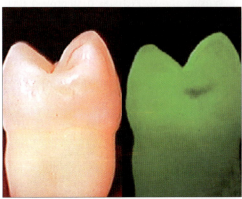

Fig. 15 Premolar before and after exposure, showing decalcified area (courtesy of Inspektor Dental Care BV, Amsterdam, NL)

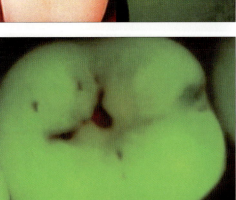

Fig. 16 Occlusal caries (courtesy of Inspektor Dental Care BV, Amsterdam, NL)

restorations, amalgam, gold, porcelain and composite, would only allow marginal caries to be detected.

New-emerging techniques in laser-assisted caries detection

Quantitative light-induced fluorescence. This is a highly sensitive method for determining short-term changes in lesions in the mouth.[43] The control unit consists of an illumination device and imaging electronics. The argon-ion laser was replaced in 1995 by a xenon-based arc-lamp and the light from this lamp is filtered by a blue-transmitting filter. A liquid light-guide transports the blue light to the teeth in the mouth and a dental mirror provides uniform illumination of the area to be recorded. The excitation wavelength around 405 nm produced by the system allows visualisation and quantification of both the dental tissues' intrinsic green fluorescence as well as the red fluorescence from bacterial origin as observed in calculus, plaque and (advanced) caries.[44,45] The green fluorescence loss observed from demineralised enamel as well as natural caries lesions is strongly correlated with mineral loss.[46-48] The red fluorescence offers insight into oral hygiene levels, allows visualisation of leaking margins of sealants and restorations[44] and is furthermore suggested for use during caries excavation.[49]

Dental calculus produces the most pronounced fluorescent intensity, carious regions produce a slightly weaker fluorescent intensity. Photo-images of this technique are given in Figures 12-16 (source www.inspektor.nl).

PS-OCT – polarisation-sensitive optical coherence tomography. Preliminary studies using OCT have proven successful at imaging hard and soft tissue in the oral cavity. Using polarisation-sensitive OCT (PS-OCT), a numerical analysis of the optical properties of the surface and subsurface enamel can be

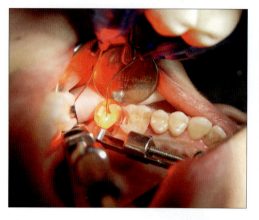
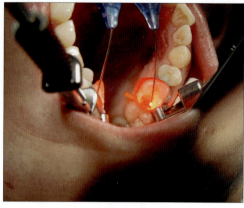

Fig. 17 (left) Photo-activated disinfection of prepared cavity, upper second molar (courtesy of T. Von Samson and Denfotex UK)

Fig. 18 (right) Photo-activated disinfection of prepared cavity, upper first molar (courtesy of T. Von Samson and Denfotex UK)

obtained. At research levels, using a near-infrared beam (λ 1,310 nm), caries detection is possible at both surface level and under composite restorations and sealants.[50,51]

Recent developments have seen the emergence of other spectroscopic analysis devices which are undergoing development, eg a blue InGaN laser diode operating at 405 nm.[52]

PHOTO-ACTIVATED DISINFECTION (PAD)

This is a development over and above the conventional use of chemicals to achieve bacterial decontamination in restorative dentistry. As opposed to chemicals that are spontaneously interactive with cellular structures, PAD employs a photo-activated liquid, a solution of tolonium chloride (a pharmaceutical grade of the vital stain toluidene blue O). Exposure of this chemical to low-level visible red light (635 nm) releases singlet oxygen that ruptures bacterial cell walls[53] (Figs 17 and 18).

During the early 1990s at the Eastman Dental Institute, London, Professors M. Wilson and G. Pearson first proved PAD killed *Streptococcus mutans*[54] in significant numbers, and reasoned that PAD could kill all bacteria involved in oral infections in caries, root canals, and periodontics,[55] thereby eliminating the most common oral infections. Research was undertaken to determine the susceptibility to photo-activated disinfection (PAD) of *Streptococcus mutans* when the organism was present in a collagen matrix[56] – an environment similar to that which would exist within a carious tooth. This research has led to the production of a commercial unit for use in dental surgery (Figs 19-22).

Recent *in vitro* and *in vivo* studies[57,58] into the use of PAD in endodontics have demonstrated the effectiveness of this therapy against a number of anaerobic bacterial strains associated with endodontic infections (*Fusobacterium nucleatum, Peptostreptococcus micros, Prevotella intermedia* and *Streptococcus intermedius*). In addition, PAD has been shown to be effective against *Enterococcus faecalis*.[59]

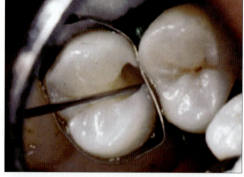
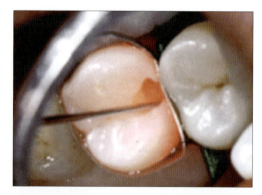

Fig. 19 (left) Laser probe in tooth cavity (courtesy of T. Von Samson and Denfotex UK)

Fig. 20 (right) Cavity decontamination (courtesy of T. Von Samson and Denfotex UK)

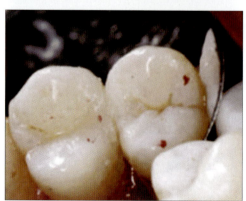
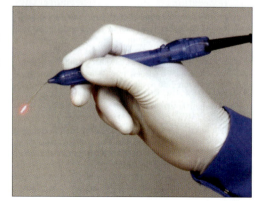

Fig. 21 (left) Completed restoration (courtesy of T. Von Samson and Denfotex UK)

Fig. 22 (right) Hand-piece and fibre. The fibre diameter equates to ISO #40 (reproduced with permission, Denfotex UK)

LASER SCANNING (ORTHODONTICS, RESTORATIVE DENTISTRY)

The development of laser-based measuring devices (eg the confocal micrometer), utilising beam-splitting of a low-energy laser and optical detector, has enabled accurate replication of the morphology of dental and oral structures and materials used in restorative dentistry.

The earliest use of laser scanning was in the field of orthodontics and facial development, to provide 3D imaging and recording of pre- and post-treatment of deformities.[60-62] Scanned data was linked to computer software using CAD (computer-assisted design).

This concept has been expanded during the last decade, to enable the scanning of restorative cavities prior to the production of cast or milled indirect restorations,[63] and the recording of oral and facial swellings.[64]

An additional associated use of laser light in oral medicine is through Raman spectroscopy. A Raman spectrum represents the scattering of incident laser light by molecular or crystal vibrations. Such vibration is quite sensitive to the molecular composition of samples being investigated, and areas of research include the *in vitro* and *in vivo* study of disease processes such as cancer, atherosclerosis and bone disease. With regard to the latter, Raman spectroscopic analysis *in vivo* of mineral and matrix changes has been shown to be useful in mapping early changes in bone tissue.[65]

Permission granted by Dr Gerry Ross, Toronto, Canada to reproduce clinical photographs, Denfotex UK in showing photo-activated disinfection and Inspektor Dental Care BV, The Netherlands for QLF information, is gratefully acknowledged.

1. Scott B. *Clinical uses of ultraviolet radiation*. GK edition. Baltimore: Stillwell, 1983.
2. Cuncliffe W J. Diseases of the skin. *Br Med J* 1973; **4:** 667-669.
3. Ennever J F. Phototherapy for neonatal jaundice. *Photochem Photobiol* 1988; **47:** 871-876.
4. Mester E, Spiry T, Szende B *et al.* Effect of laser rays on wound healing. *Am J Surg* 1971; **122:** 532-535.
5. Wolbarsht M L (ed). *Clinical aspects of laser research*. pp 116. New York: Plenum Press, 1977.
6. Torabinejad M, Mindroiu T, Bakland L. Detection of kinins in human periapical lesions. *J Dent Res* 1989; **68:** 201.
7. Passarella S. Increase of proton electrochemical potential and ATP synthesis in rat liver mitochondria irradiated in vitro by helium-neon laser. *FEBS Lett* 1984; **175:** 95-99.
8. Karu T. Photobiological fundamentals of low powered laser therapy. *IEEE J Quantum Electron* 1987; **23:** 1703-1717.
9. Dube A, Bansal H, Gupta P K. Modulation of macrophage structure and function by low level He-Ne laser irradiation. *Photochem Photobiol Sci* 2003; **2:** 851-855.
10. Stadler I, Evans R, Kolb B *et al*. In vitro effects of low-level laser irradiation at 660 nm on peripheral blood lymphocytes. *Lasers Surg Med* 2000; **27:** 255-261.
11. Kreisler M, Christoffers A B, Willershausen B, d'Hoedt B. Effect of low-level GaAlAs laser irradiation on the proliferation rate of human periodontal ligament fibroblasts: an in vitro study. *J Clin Periodontol* 2003; **30:** 353-358.
12. Kovacs I B, Mester E, Gorog P. Stimulation of wound healing with laser beam in the rat. *Experientia* 1974; **30:** 1275-1276.
13. Enwemeka C S, Parker J C, Dowdy D S, Harkness E E, Sanford L E, Woodruff L D. The efficacy of low-power lasers in tissue repair and pain control: a meta-analysis study. *Photomed Laser Surg* 2004; **22:** 323-329.
14. Honmura A. Therapeutic effect of GaAlAs diode laser irradiation on experimentally induced inflammation in rats. *Lasers Surg Med* 1992; **12:** 441-449.
15. Laakso E L, Cramond T, Richardson C, Galligan J P. Plasma ACTH and β-endorphin levels in response to low level laser therapy for myofascial trigger points. *Laser Ther* 1994; **3:** 133-142.
16. Montesinos M. Experimental effects of low power laser in encephalon and endorphin synthesis. *J Eur Med Laser Assoc* 1988; **1:** 2-7.
17. Schultz H. Ueber hefegifte. *Pflugers Archiv fur die gesamte Physiologie des Menschen und der Tierre* 1888; **42:** 517-541.
18. Al-Watban. Effect of HeNe laser and Polygen on CHO cells. *J Clin Laser Surg Med* 2000; **18:** 145-150.
19. Takata A N, Zaneveld L, Richter W. Laser-induced thermal damage in skin. *Aerospace Med Rep* 1977; Rep. SAM-TR-77-38.
20. Bjordal J M, Couppe, C, Ljunggren A. Low level laser therapy for tendinopathies; evidence of a dose-related pattern. *Phys Ther Reviews* 2001; **6:** 91-100.
21. Kimura Y, Wilder-Smith P, Yonaga K, Matsumoto K. Treatment of dentine hypersensitivity by laser; a review. *J Clin Periodontol* 2000; **27:** 715-721.
22. Taube S, Piironen J, Ylipaavalniemi P. Helium-neon laser therapy in the prevention of post-operative swelling and pain after wisdom tooth extraction. *Proc Finn Dent Soc* 1990; **86:** 23-27.
23. Vélez-González M, Urrea-Arbaláes A, Serra-Baldrich E, Pavesi M, Camarasa J M, Trelles M A. Treatment of relapse in herpes simplex on labia and facial areas and of primary herpes simplex on genital areas and "area pudenda" with low power HeNe laser or acyclovir administered orally. *Proc SPIE* 1995; **2630:** 43-50.
24. Schindl A, Neuman R. Low intensity laser therapy is an effective treatment for recurrent herpes simplex infection: results from a randomised double-blind placebo controlled study. *J Invest Dermatol* 1999; **113:** 221-223.
25. Pinheiro A L, Cavalcanti E T, Pinheiro T I, Alves M J, Manzi C T. Low-level laser therapy in the management of disorders of the maxillofacial region. *J Clin Laser Med Surg* 1997; **15:** 181-183.
26. Howell R M, Cohen D M, Powell G L, Green J G. The use of low energy laser therapy to treat aphthous ulcers. *Ann Dent* 1988; **47:** 16-18.
27. Wong S F, Wilder-Smith P. Pilot study of laser effects on oral mucositis in patients receiving chemotherapy. *Cancer J* 2002; **8:** 247-254.
28. Wilder-Smith P. The soft laser; therapeutic tool or popular placebo? *Oral Surg Oral Med Oral Pathol* 1988; **66:** 654-658.
29. Kelsey W P, Blankenau R J, Powell G L, Barkmeier W W, Stormberg E F. Power and time requirements for use of the argon laser to polymerize composite resins. *J Clin Laser Med Surg* 1992; **10:** 273-278.
30. Talbot T Q, Blankenau R J, Zobitz M E, Weaver A L, Lohse C M, Rebellato J. Effect of argon laser irradiation on shear bond strength of orthodontic brackets: an in vitro study. *Am J Orthod Dentofac Orthop* 2000; **118:** 274-279.
31. Powell G L, Blankenau R J. Effects of argon laser curing on dentin shear bond strengths. *J Clin Laser Med Surg* 1996; **14:** 111-113.
32. Blankenau R J, Kelsey W P, Powell G L, Shearer G O, Barkmeier W W, Cavel W T. Degree of composite resin polymerization with visible light and argon laser. *Am J Dent* 1991; **4:** 40-42.
33. Bjelkhagen H, Sundström F. A clinically applicable laser luminescence method for the early detection of dental caries. *IEEE J Quantum Electron* 1981; **17:** 266-270.
34. Bjelkhagen H, Sundström F, Angmar-Månsson B, Ryden H. Early detection of enamel caries by the luminescence excited by visible laser light. *Swed Dent J* 1982; **6:** 1-7.
35. Hafström-Björkman U, Sundström F, de Josselin de Jong E, Oliveby A, Angmar-Månsson B. Comparison of laser fluorescence and longitudinal microradiography for quantitative assessment of in vitro enamel caries. *Caries Res* 1992; **26:** 241-247.
36. de Josselin de Jong E, Sundström F, Westerling H, Tranaeus S, ten Bosch J J, Angmar-Månsson B. A new method for in vivo quantification of changes in initial enamel caries with laser fluorescence. *Caries Res* 1995; **29:** 2-7.
37. König K, Hibst R, Meyer H, Flemming G, Schneckenburger H. Laser-induced autofluorescence of carious regions of human teeth and caries-involved bacteria. *Proc SPIE* 1993; **2080:** 170-180.

38. Dolowy W C, Brandes M L, Gouterman M, Parker J D, Lind J. Fluorescence of dental calculus from cats, dogs, and humans and of bacteria cultured from dental calculus. *J Vet Dent* 1995; **12:** 105-109.
39. Hibst R, Gall R. Development of a diode laser-based fluorescence detector. *Caries Res* 1998; **32:** 294.
40. Hibst R, Paulus R. Caries detection by red excited fluorescence: investigations on fluorophores. *Caries Res* 1999; **33:** 295.
41. Lussi A, Megert B, Longbottom C, Reich E, Francescut P. Clinical performance of a laser fluorescence device for detection of occlusal caries lesions. *Eur J Oral Sci* 2001; **109:** 14-19.
42. Bader J D, Shugars D A. A systematic review of the performance of a laser fluorescence device for detecting caries. *J Am Dent Assoc* 2004; **135:** 1413-1426.
43. Stookey G K. Optical methods – quantitative light fluorescence. *J Dent Res* 2004; **83 (Suppl):** C84-C88.
44. Heinrich-Weltzien R, Kühnisch J, van der Veen M, de Josselin de Jong E, Stosser L. Quantitative light-induced fluorescence (QLF) – a potential method for the dental practitioner. *Quintessence Int* 2003; **34:** 181-188.
45. van der Veen M H, Buchalla W, de Josselin de Jong E. QLF™ technologies: recent advances. *In* Stookey G K (ed) *Early detection of dental caries III: proceedings of the 6th Indiana conference.* pp 291-304. Indianapolis: Indiana University School of Dentistry, 2003.
46. Hafström-Björkman U, Sundström F, de Josselin de Jong E, Oliveby A, Angmar-Månsson B. Comparison of laser fluorescence and longitudinal microradiography for quantitative assessment of in vitro enamel caries. *Caries Res* 1992; **26:** 241-247.
47. Emami Z, Al-Khateeb S, de Josselin de Jong E, Sundström F, Trollsås K, Angmar-Månsson B. Mineral loss in incipient caries lesions quantified with laser fluorescence and longitudinal microradiography. A methodologic study. *Acta Odontol Scand* 1996; **54:** 8-13.
48. Ando M, van Der Veen M H, Schemehorn B R, Stookey G K. Comparative study to quantify demineralized enamel in deciduous and permanent teeth using laser- and light-induced fluorescence techniques. *Caries Res* 2001; **35:** 464-470.
49. Lennon A M, Buchalla W, Switalski L, Stookey G K. Residual caries detection using visible fluorescence. *Caries Res* 2002; **36:** 315-319.
50. Fried D, Xie J, Shafi S, Featherstone J D, Breunig T M, Le C. Imaging caries lesions and lesion progression with polarization sensitive optical coherence tomography. *J Biomed Opt* 2002; **7:** 618-627.
51. Jones R S, Staninec M, Fried D. Imaging artificial caries under composite sealants and restorations. *J Biomed Opt* 2004; **9:** 1297-1304.
52. Ribeiro A, Rousseau C, Girkin J *et al.* A preliminary investigation of a spectroscopic technique for the diagnosis of natural caries lesions. *J Dent* 2005; **33:** 73-78.
53. Soukos N S, Wilson M, Burns T, Speight P M. The photodynamic effects of toluidine blue on human oral keratinocytes and fibroblasts and Streptococcus sanguis evaluated in vitro. *Lasers Surg Med* 1996; **18:** 253-259.
54. Burns T, Wilson M, Pearson G J. Sensitisation of cariogenic bacteria to killing by light from a helium/neon laser. *Med Microbiol* 1993; **38:** 401-405.
55. Wilson M, Dobson J, Harvey W. Sensitisation of oral bacteria to killing by low-power laser radiation. *Current Microbiol* 1992; **25:** 77-81.
56. Williams J A, Pearson G J, Colles M J, Wilson M. The photo-activated antibacterial action of toluidine blue O in a collagen matrix and in carious dentine. *Caries Res* 2004; **38:** 530-536.
57. Williams J A, Pearson G J, John Colles M. Antibacterial action of photoactivated disinfection {PAD} used on endodontic bacteria in planktonic suspension and in artificial and human root canals. *J Dent* 2006; **34:** 363-371.
58. Bonsor S J, Nichol R, Reid T M, Pearson G J. Microbiological evaluation of photo-activated disinfection in endodontics (an *in vivo* study). *Br Dent J* 2006; **200:** 337-341.
59. Lee M T, Bird P S, Walsh L J. Photo-activated disinfection of root canals: a new role for lasers in endodontics. *Austr Endod J* 2004; **30:** 93-98.
60. McCance A M, Moss J P, Wright W R, Linney A D, James D R. A three-dimensional soft tissue analysis of 16 skeletal Class III patients following bimaxillary surgery. *Br J Oral Maxillofac Surg* 1992; **30:** 221-232.
61. McCance A M, Moss J P, Fright W R, James D R, Linney A D. A three dimensional analysis of soft and hard tissue changes following bimaxillary orthognathic surgery in skeletal III patients. *Br J Oral Maxillofac Surg* 1992; **30:** 305-312.
62. Commer P, Bourauel C, Maier K, Jager A. Construction and testing of a computer-based intraoral laser scanner for determining tooth positions. *Med Eng Phys* 2000; **22:** 625-635.
63. Denissen H W, van der Zel J M, van Waas M A. Measurement of the margins of partial-coverage tooth preparations for CAD/CAM. *Int J Prosthodont* 1999; **12:** 395-400.
64. Harrison J A, Nixon M A, Fright W R, Snape L. Use of hand-held laser scanning in the assessment of facial swelling: a preliminary study. *Br J Oral Maxillofac Surg* 2004; **42:** 8-17.
65. Tarnowski C P, Ignelzi M A Jr, Wang W, Taboas J M, Goldstein S A, Morris M D. Earliest mineral and matrix changes in force-induced musculoskeletal disease as revealed by Raman microspectroscopic imaging. *J Bone Miner Res* 2004; **19:** 64-71.

IN BRIEF

- A range of 'loose' (non-bound to the muco-periosteal complex) soft tissue pathologies are amenable to treatment with surgical lasers.
- Laser-assisted surgery should follow strict guidelines of 'best practice' approach, as employed in conventional therapies.
- Laser-assisted surgical sites heal by secondary intention.
- In comparison to scalpel incisions, laser cutting heals no faster, but may be more predictable through the control of bleeding and bacterial contamination.

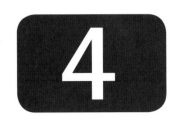

Lasers and soft tissue: 'loose' soft tissue surgery

Oral soft tissue is composed of collagen, water, pigmented connective tissue, blood and lymphatic vessels. In that each may be considered target chromophores, all commercially available laser wavelengths in dentistry will interact with these component elements to a greater or lesser extent. What is of prime importance is that consideration is given to the predominant chromophore in any target tissue and the laser wavelength matched to achieve maximum absorption of light energy. Laser surgery can offer haemostasis, fewer post-operative complications and greater patient acceptance. This chapter examines the common 'loose' soft tissue management procedures in general dental practice and how the use of lasers can enable the clinician to deliver responsible care.

LASERS IN DENTISTRY

1. Introduction, history of lasers and laser light production
2. Laser-tissue interaction
3. Low-level laser use in dentistry
4. **Lasers and soft tissue: 'loose' soft tissue surgery**
5. Lasers and soft tissue: 'fixed' soft tissue surgery
6. Lasers and soft tissue: periodontal therapy
7. Surgical laser use in implantology and endodontics
8. Surgical lasers and hard dental tissue
9. Laser regulation and safety in general dental practice

BIOLOGICAL CONSIDERATIONS

In an otherwise healthy individual, the biological mechanisms that allow healing to take place will always follow the same pathways, irrespective of whether tissue injury is due to a scalpel, thermal, chemical or traumatic cause. Consolidation of wound protection – blood clotting and plasma retention, elimination of bacterial infection and other aspects of classical inflammatory response – is followed by an in-growth of epithelial and endothelial cell types, which then proceeds to maturation of wound healing over time. Any potential for scar tissue formation can be affected by the type of tissue, presence of tissue mediators and growth factors, the cause of the wound, whether healing is by primary or secondary intention and, occasionally, racial type.[1,2]

In an ideal situation, the post surgical healing will be such as to restore stability, form and function to the tissue. In oral soft tissue surgery, where appropriate, the aesthetics of the tissue will be maintained or, as is often the desired outcome, improved with regard to fixed restorations.

Whenever soft tissue is incised using a scalpel, there will a succession of events that will dictate tissue management:

(i) **Bleeding:** most intra-oral soft tissue procedures associated with general dental practice would normally involve the cutting or puncture of small-diameter vessels (arterioles, venules and capillaries)

(ii) **Dressings:** the aim of any dressing will be to arrest bleeding and allow clot formation, stabilise the cut margin, stabilise tissue to allow healing and prevent possible disturbance of the incision

(iii) **Contamination:** the ingress of bacteria into the incision site, sutures and dressings is inevitable and will act to compromise the inflammatory response. This will often add to any post-operative pain or discomfort

(iv) **Short-term follow-up:** removal of sutures and/or dressings

(v) **Long-term:** re-organisation of epithelial and endothelial component structure with possible shrinkage.

Assuming correct laser wavelength per tissue site and appropriate power parameters, the healing of oral soft tissue is often termed 'uneventful'. Often, if not always, the need for dressings or sutures is avoided. Irrespective of the wavelength, all soft tissue healing will be by secondary intention, in that it will be impossible to oppose the cut tissue edges to their original alignment. Of note, however,

LASERS IN DENTISTRY

Fig. 1 (left) Fibroma, lateral border of tongue

Fig. 2 (right) Nd:YAG laser excision – 320 μm fibre non-contact, 250 mJ/15 Hz, average power 3.75 W

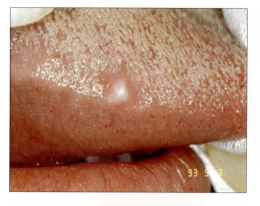
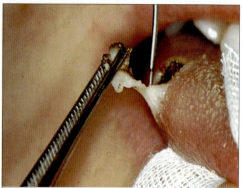

Fig. 3 (left) Immediately post-operative, showing peripheral zone of oedema

Fig. 4 (right) Three days post-operative, showing hydration of coagulum

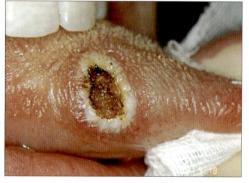
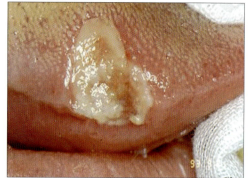

Fig. 5 (left) Post-operative healing at two weeks

Fig. 6 (right) Fibroma, left oral commisure

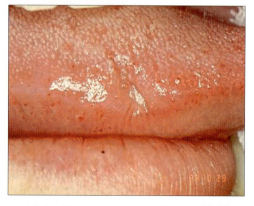
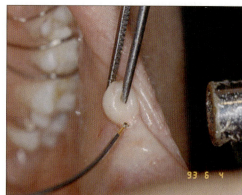

Fig. 7 (left) Nd:YAG laser beam directed into 'discard'

Fig. 8 (right) Immediately post-operative

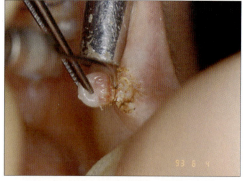
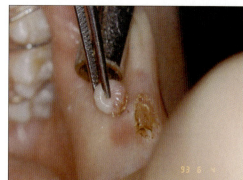

Fig. 9 (left) Healing at 10 days

Fig. 10 (right) Fibroma, buccal mucosa

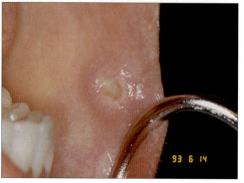
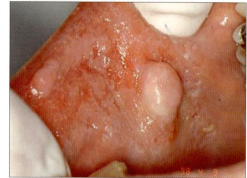

SOFT TISSUES LOOSE

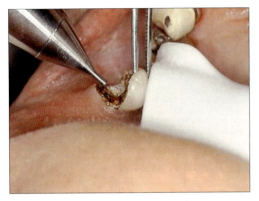
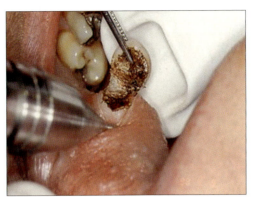

Fig. 11 (left) CO_2 laser excision. The high-speed suction is positioned to remove ablation products, cool the tissue and prevent distant, non-target laser-tissue interaction

Fig. 12 (right) Haemostasis achieved

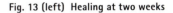

Fig. 13 (left) Healing at two weeks

is the phenomenon of lack of post-incisional contamination by bacteria, due to a possible sterility of the cut surface,[3] but certainly through the protective layer of coagulum of plasma and blood products – a tenacious film that allows early healing to take place underneath.[4] Additionally, studies with longer wavelengths show that there is a lack of fibroblast alignment associated with the incision line and consequent reduced tissue shrinkage through scarring.[5] Such findings are often borne out in the clinical setting.

SURGICAL CONSIDERATIONS

The use of a laser, as with more conventional instruments, demands of the clinician basic surgical skills which should remain paramount. Knowledge of the anatomical site, sound diagnostic skills, appreciation of the desired post-surgical outcome and functional needs should be combined with a thorough understanding of the patient's dental and medical history. Where appropriate, the nature of any pathology should be assessed prior to surgical intervention and referral protocols for specialist care should apply, if necessary.

'LOOSE' SOFT TISSUE SURGERY

Within general dental practice, this would include the removal of fibromata, mucocoele, small haemangiomata, denture granulomata, labial and lingual fraenectomies and treatment of non-erosive lichen planus and mucocytosis.

The aetiology of the lesion should be assessed, together with an understanding of the tissue composition. As with a scalpel, the abnormal tissue, if possible, should be placed under tension to allow accurate cleavage. In most cases, the laser hand-piece tip is held in close approximation to, and just out of contact with, the tissue surface. In this way, the laser energy is allowed to effect the incision and minimise the build-up of debris on the tip, which can distort the laser-tissue interaction.

As was seen in previous chapters in this book, 'safe' soft tissue cleavage, avoiding the potential of collateral thermal damage, is related to correct wavelength/tissue assessment, minimum laser power to achieve tissue cleavage and thermal relaxation measures to prevent heat build-up. Shorter laser wavelengths (diode, 810, 980 nm; Nd:YAG, 1,064 nm) transverse the epithelium and penetrate two to six millimetres into the tissue, whereas longer wavelengths have minimal penetration. As surgical cutting proceeds, the heat generated seals small blood and lymphatic vessels, reducing or eliminating bleeding and oedema. Denatured proteins within tissue and plasma give rise to a surface zone of a tenacious layer, termed 'coagulum' or 'char', which serves to protect the surgical wound from frictional or bacterial action. Clinically, during 48-72 hours post-surgery, this layer undergoes hydration from saliva, swells and disintegrates and eventually is lost to reveal an early healing bed of new tissue. This sequence of events can be seen in the removal of a lingual fibroma using a Nd:YAG laser. The area of reactive tissue oedema surrounding the ablation site indicates the penetrating conductive heat effects found with shorter wavelength lasers, such as the Nd:YAG (Figs 1-5).

This risk of collateral thermal damage can be minimised by directing the laser beam into the discard tissue (Figs 6-9).

With longer wavelengths (Er,Cr:YSGG, 2,780 nm; Er:YAG, 2,940 nm; CO_2, 10,600 nm), the risk of deep penetration is minimised and surgical incisions can be deemed less potentially damaging. However, in the author's experience, the spot size of most CO_2 lasers is larger than the fibre optic-delivered shorter wavelengths and hand-piece tips used with erbium lasers, which renders incisions with CO_2 wavelength potentially less accurate. This has little consequence in 'loose' soft tissue surgery, but may have an effect in

LASERS IN DENTISTRY

Fig. 14 (left) Traumatic haemangioma

Fig. 15 (right) Use of diode (810 nm) laser. Note red aiming beam to assist targeting of infrared laser beam

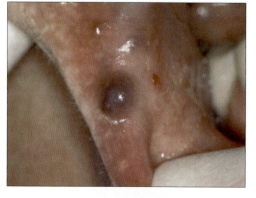
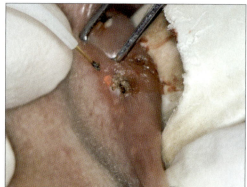

Fig. 16 (left) Immediately post-operative

Fig. 17 (right) Healing at two weeks

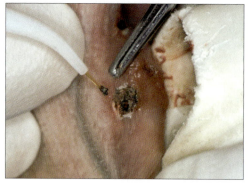
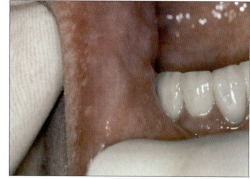

Fig. 18 Lower labial fraenectomy using Nd:YAG laser at excessive power levels (5.0 W average power), where underlying bone damage occurred

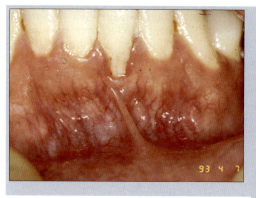
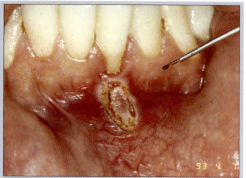
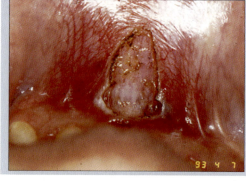

detailed surgery, where aesthetics are a prime consideration (Figs 10-13).

Shorter, visible and near-infrared wavelengths are readily absorbed by pigmented tissue. This can be used advantageously in the treatment of small haemangiomata, especially those of possible traumatic origin (Figs 14-17).

LASER FLUENCE LEVELS AND SURGICAL INCISIONS

The objective of correct ('safe') laser energy per surgical site (fluence – energy density – J/cm^2) shall be to use the minimum level, commensurate with the desired effect.

Insufficient laser energy levels may not initiate tissue ablation, whereas excessive levels can lead to carbonisation and possible deep collateral thermal damage. Carbon, whether present as a build-up on a fibre tip or tissue surface, absorbs all light wavelengths and quickly over-heats. This becomes a source of secondary thermal energy and acts as a 'branding iron', leading to conductive thermal damage.

For most intra-oral minor surgical procedures, an average laser power (J/s) setting should be in the range of two to four Watts. This is based on personal experience and recommended levels found in manufacturers' user manuals. Whilst this might be easy to comprehend in those continuous-wave (CW) emission lasers (diode 810-980 nm and CO_2), where the machine panel display is the average power output, for those free-running (FRP) lasers where energy per pulse and pulse numbers are displayed, the average power is the product of these values (eg 200 mJ per pulse/15 pulses

SOFT TISSUES LOOSE

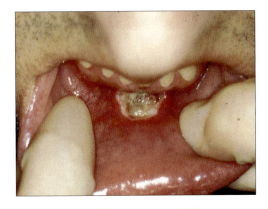
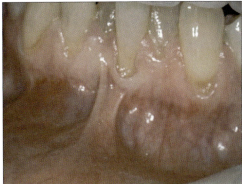

Fig. 19 (left) Post-operative tissue necrosis

Fig. 20 (right) High fraenal attachment

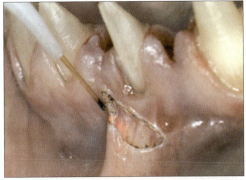
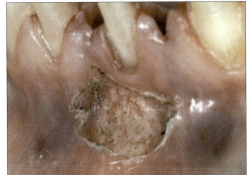

Fig. 21 (left) Nd:YAG laser beam angled correctly, 2.5 W average power

Fig. 22 (right) Immediately post-operative

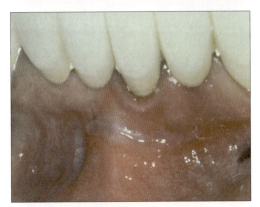
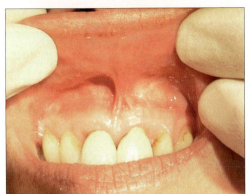

Fig. 23 (left) Healing at three weeks post-operative

Fig. 24 (right) 'Failed' scalpel fraenectomy

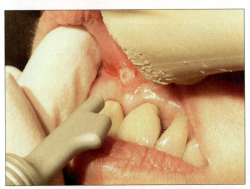
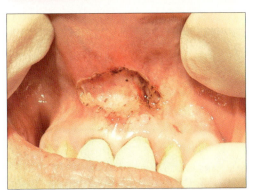

Fig. 25 (left) Er:YAG laser in use

Fig. 26 (right) Immediately post-operative

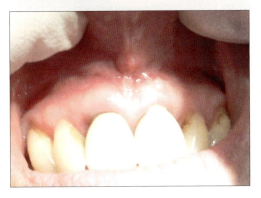
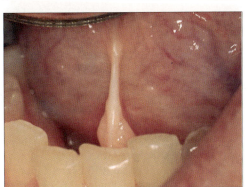

Fig. 27 (left) Healing at four weeks

Fig. 28 (right) Restrictive lingual fraenum

LASERS IN DENTISTRY

Fig. 29 (left) Immediately post-operative. Diode laser

Fig. 30 (right) Healing at three weeks

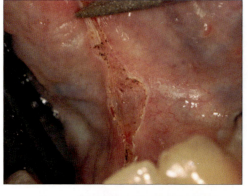 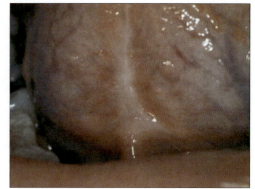

Fig. 31 (left) Benign non-erosive lichen planus

Fig. 32 (right) 'Laser peel' using CO_2 laser in de-focussed mode

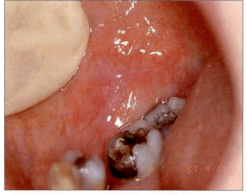 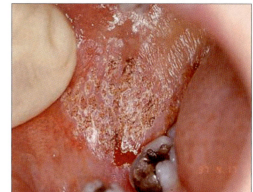

Fig. 33 (left) Healing at one month

Fig. 34 (right) 'Denture granuloma' associated with edentulous lower ridge

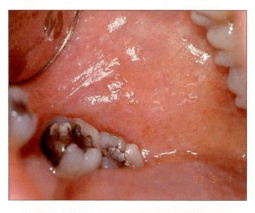 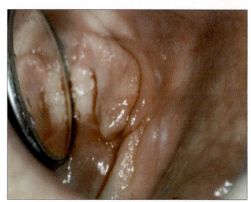

Fig. 35 (left) Laser excision of excess tissue (diode 810 nm, 320 μm fibre, 1.7 W CW). Due to potential penetration of the beam, the beam is angled into 'discard' tissue

Fig. 36 (right) Traction aids tissue cleavage. Correct power values reduce carbonisation

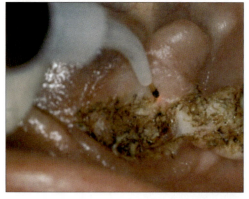 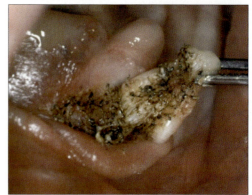

per s = 3.5 W average power). With regard to the latter, increasing the value of pulses will reduce the thermal relaxation potential. This is less of a problem with longer FRP wavelengths, eg Er:YAG and Er,Cr:YSGG, due to their shallow penetration, and does indeed allow better coagulative capabilities for these wavelengths with pigmented tissue.

Intrinsically linked to the average power is the close location of anatomical sites that might be damaged through excessive power values[6] (Figs 18 and 19). In this case, the penetration of the near-infrared wavelength beam was sufficient to cause thermal damage to the underlying periosteum and bone, resulting in tissue necrosis and a disfiguring cleft in the overlying attached gingiva.

This disastrous result can be compared with a similar procedure, where the same wavelength is used at lower average power values

SOFT TISSUES LOOSE

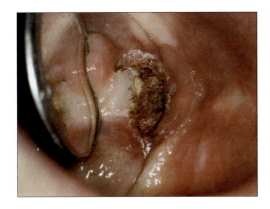 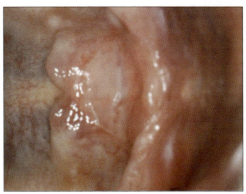

Fig. 37 (left) Immediately post-operative, no dressings required

Fig. 38 (right) Healing at two weeks

(2.5 W), the laser beam is kept parallel to and away from the underlying bone and sufficient time intervals employed to allow tissue cooling (Figs 20-23).

Wherever possible, 'loose' soft tissue incisions can be accomplished more easily if the site is placed under tension. One of the commonest procedures where laser use might be deemed superior to scalpel is the fraenectomy. As with all laser soft tissue surgery, it is essential to appreciate that it is the light energy that is effecting the incision. Using a light 'brush stroke' action, with the delivery tip just out of contact and the tissue under tension, the tissue is seen to 'melt' away. The absence of bleeding significantly reduces post-operative swelling and discomfort and the absence of sutures can minimise the risk of distortion of anatomy. Figures 24-27 show a case where a revision surgery of a 'failed' scalpel fraenectomy results in a more acceptable result. The Er:YAG laser is readily absorbed by the fibrous scar tissue. Figures 28-30 show a case of a lingual fraenectomy, on a 15 year-old patient, using a diode (810 nm) laser.

Where flat surface pathology requires excision, the minimal penetration of the CO_2 laser wavelength can be used to advantage in performing a 'laser peel'. This requires a 'de-focussed' or long non-contact technique, to prevent incisional-type cutting. The 'char' layer produced with this technique is removed with damp gauze, allowing the procedure to be completed to the desired depth. Lesions such as non-erosive lichen planus, where specialist referral and biopsy have endorsed a benign diagnosis, can be treated successfully with minimal distortion of anatomical structures (Figs 31-33).

Another clinical situation where gross tissue removal makes haemostasis, bacterial control and dressings difficult, could be the removal of hyperplastic 'denture' granulomata. As Figures 34-38 show, the use of a laser (diode 810 nm in this case) allows tissue excision, management and healing to be accomplished with minimum disruption.

SUMMARY

An overview has been given of the interaction of laser light with 'loose' soft tissue structures in the mouth. The advantages of this modality in the approach to surgery have been given, together with the need to match laser energy levels and absorption potential with surgical technique and appropriate patient management.

1. Bayat A, Arscott G, Ollier W E, McGrouther D A, Ferguson M W. Keloid disease: clinical relevance of single versus multiple site scars. *Br J Plast Surg* 2005; **58:** 28-37.
2. Funato N, Moriyama K, Baba Y, Kuroda T. Evidence for apoptosis induction in myofibroblasts during palatal mucoperiosteal repair. *J Dent Res* 1999; **78:** 1511-1517.
3. Kaminer R, Liebow C, Margarone J E 3rd, Zambon J J. Bacteremia following laser and conventional surgery in hamsters. *J Oral Maxillofac Surg* 1990; **48:** 45-48.
4. Nanami T, Shiba H, Ikeuchi S, Nagai T, Asanami S, Shibata T. Clinical applications and basic studies of laser in dentistry and oral surgery. *Keio J Med* 1993; **42:** 199-201.
5. Fisher S E, Frame J W, Browne R M, Tranter R M. A comparative histological study of wound healing following CO_2 laser and conventional surgical excision of canine buccal mucosa. *Arch Oral Biol* 1983; **28:** 287-291.
6. Spencer P, Cobb C M, Wieliczka D M, Glaros A G, Morris P J. Change in temperature of subjacent bone during soft tissue laser ablation. *J Periodontol* 1998; **69:** 1278-1282.

IN BRIEF

- Lasers can be used in the surgical management of gingival hyperplasias, tooth exposure and hyperpigmentation.
- Precise excision of gingival tissue relative to restorative procedures, with associated haemostatic control, can often allow treatment to proceed more smoothly and quickly.
- Care should be observed when using lasers in areas where there is a close approximation of various hard and soft tissues, to avoid unwanted thermal damage.

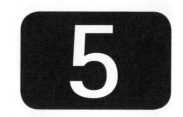

Lasers and soft tissue: 'fixed' soft tissue surgery

Within a general practice setting, there are few benign pathological conditions of the attached or keratinised gingival complex that are not amenable to simple surgical intervention. The majority of surgical procedures are adjunctive to the delivery of restorative dentistry. There is an understandable dogma worldwide towards the management of soft tissues as they interface with restorative procedures. Contemporary teaching, both at undergraduate and postgraduate level, would recognise the need for a period of wound healing and stability, based on scalpel-induced incisional therapy. The use of laser wavelengths, based on predictable evidence-based protocols, has re-defined the surgical management of keratinised mucosa that is bound to the underlying periosteum and bone. This can be seen as being of benefit to the clinician in determining the outcome, and the patient in achieving quality results.

LASERS IN DENTISTRY

1. Introduction, history of lasers and laser light production
2. Laser-tissue interaction
3. Low-level laser use in dentistry
4. Lasers and soft tissue: 'loose' soft tissue surgery
5. **Lasers and soft tissue: 'fixed' soft tissue surgery**
6. Lasers and soft tissue: periodontal therapy
7. Surgical laser use in implantology and endodontics
8. Surgical lasers and hard dental tissue
9. Laser regulation and safety in general dental practice

SURGICAL PROCEDURES

The range of benign pathology affecting the muco-periosteal tissue of the dento-alveolar complex includes the following:
- Epulis
- Giant cell granuloma
- Inflammatory and drug-induced gingival hyperplasia
- Tooth exposure
- Melanin removal.

In addition, there is a range of gingival adaptation procedures, both to allow restorative procedures and to allow access to restorative margins during restorative procedures.

When used correctly, laser energy will act primarily as a means of incision, excision or ablation. Its advantage over the scalpel is the avoidance of bleeding, dressings and sutures and lowered potential for post-operative bacterial contamination. The use of a laser should neither supplant nor compromise a sound approach to surgical technique or correct patient management. Wherever appropriate, laser surgery in and around the gingival cuff should seek to preserve a biological width, ie the zones of connective and epithelial tissues attached to the tooth, minimum 3 mm in depth, that maintains alveolar bone height, gingival margin stability and health and prevents overgrowth.[1-3]

LASER-TISSUE INTERACTION AND KERATINISED MUCOSA – RISK ANALYSIS

As discussed before, the prime interactive mechanism is photothermal, ie incident laser energy is absorbed by target chromophores and converted to heat, which effects tissue change. With shorter wavelengths (diode, Nd:YAG), there is risk of deeper penetration of the light energy. With longer wavelengths (Er,Cr:YSGG, Er:YAG and CO_2), tissue penetration is considerably less, but there is potential for the build-up of char (carbonised products of ablation). Keratinised mucosa overlying the alveolar ridge exists as an outer epithelium layer and an inner connective tissue layer, separated by the basal lamina, in thickness from 0.5-4.0 mm.[4] The underlying periosteum and bone, together with root surface at gingival margin levels, can be susceptible to thermal damage. This risk can exist through the penetration of short wavelengths or the conductive heat effects arising from long wavelength char that is super-heated.[5-9]

It is advisable, therefore, to assess the thickness, vascularity and position of any target

SOFT TISSUES FIXED

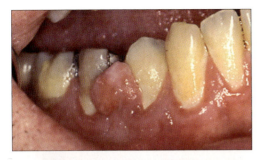

Fig. 1 Giant cell granuloma at LR 4,5

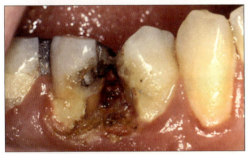

Fig. 2 Immediately post-laser excision

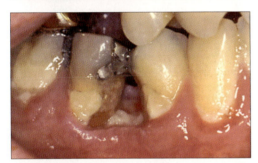

Fig. 3 Sequestrum two weeks post-operative

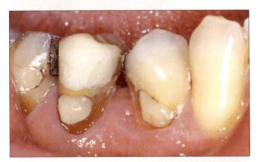

Fig. 4 10 years follow-up

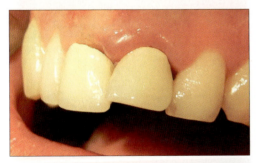

Fig. 5 Pre-treatment

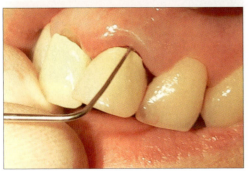

Fig. 6 Tissue assessment

gingival tissue, together with an appraisal of adjacent bone and tooth tissue.

Post-ablation tissue should be discarded, either through the use of a curette or damp cotton wool or gauze, to minimise the build-up of carbonised debris.

Figures 1-4 demonstrate the risk of deep penetration of a near-infrared Nd:YAG laser wavelength[6,10-12] during the removal of a giant cell granuloma. Laser therapy has been cited as a possible modality in treating this condition.[13] A perceived need to remove all granulomatous tissue resulted in the (erroneous) choice of excessive power values (>5.0 Watts average power). Not only did it become evident through uncharacteristic post-operative pain that too much power had been used, but also, within a few weeks, a bone sequestrum appeared. In addition, within a year, the tooth required root-canal therapy, possibly due to transmitted laser energy. Thankfully, the patient accepted the consequences with good grace and the soft tissue complex regained its integrity and stability through the ensuing 10 years.

A comparison of laser-tissue interaction between two differing wavelengths, illustrating expected and unwanted effects, is shown in Figures 5-13. This involved the removal of free-gingival tissue, commensurate with biological width, prior to placement of new crowns at UL1, UR1. The increased vascularity of the left gingival tissue prompted the use of a pigment-absorbed laser wavelength[14] (diode 810 nm), whereas the right gingival tissue, of a more normal consistency, merited the use of a CO_2 wavelength.[15]

As is often seen, the use of near-infrared wavelength laser energy results in desiccation and fragmentation of tissue, which can be removed with a sharp curette. Comparatively, the longer CO_2 laser, used in a slightly non-contact mode, gives rise to a wider zone of ablation and a less accurate incision line due to beam divergence.[16] In this case, it is evident that the tooth tissue has been exposed to the laser energy, resulting in a 'white area' of surface interaction.[17] The tooth would be subsequently prepared for restoration and the disrupted tooth surface removed.

In order to protect the adjacent, or underlying, tooth tissue, a non-reflective, non absorbent instrument can be positioned within the gingival sulcus.[18]

LASER EXCISION OF BENIGN PATHOLOGY

To perform a laser procedure properly, the surgeon uses the laser with the correct wavelength and selects the appropriate fluence and exposure time to achieve a selective photothermolytic, photomechanical or photochemical effect on the target. In earlier chapters in this book, the assessment of average power was explained and, with regard to the photothermolytic interaction, due regard should be given to thermal relaxation in order to

LASERS IN DENTISTRY

Fig. 7 Diode laser excision

Fig. 8 Removal of discard tissue with curette

Fig. 9 Adherent discard attached to optic fibre

Fig. 10 Use of CO_2 laser at UR 1

Fig. 11 Discard tissue. Note wider incision width

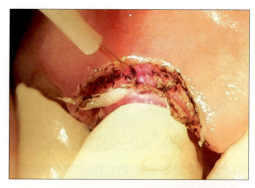
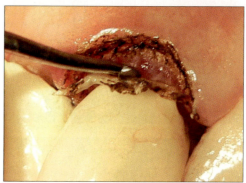
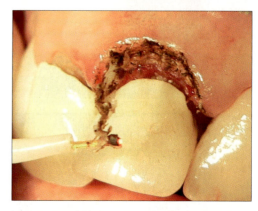
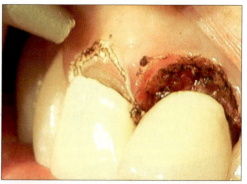
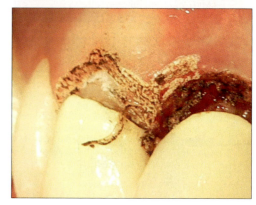

minimise unwanted effects. Laser power levels of 1.5-3.0 Watts with intervals are considered sufficient for most, if not all gingival procedures. With free-running pulsed (FRP) deliveries, shorter pulse-widths will produce higher peak values and ablate faster, but risk collateral damage; higher numbers of pulses per second, even coupled with low energy-per-pulse values, will result in less thermal relaxation. It is considered good practice with all wavelengths to select a low energy level at first, or to approach the tissue in a de-focussed mode, to assess the level of interaction.

With simple hyperplasia, wherever possible, the laser beam should be directed into the discard tissue and excision completed in a careful and deliberate manner (Figs 14-17).

With a more pedunculated epulis, it should be possible to aid excision by placing the lesion under tension. Aetiological factors should obviously be addressed to prevent recurrence (Figs 18-21).

The use of lasers to treat drug-induced gingival hyperplasia has been advocated through several studies. This can be of great assistance where either the general medical condition merits a simple surgical procedure, or the underlying blood-picture is compromised.[19-23] The associated cervical caries arising from limited access can be treated concurrently, due to the ability to control soft tissue bleeding (Figs 22-25).

The facility to combine soft tissue management with hard tissue treatment is a major benefit of laser use, when compared to more conventional therapy. Not only does this represent considerable benefit to the practitioner, but the patient management is deemed less complicated, as appointments can be condensed and sutures and dressing packs avoided. Very often, a tooth fracture, otherwise committed to extraction, can be treated and restored successfully, resulting in many more years of function. The often-achieved phenomenon of stability of the post-surgical gingival margin can be utilised in achieving good aesthetic results (Figs 26-29).

Where the fracture has extended below the alveolar bone margin, or where the biologic width might be compromised, the safe ablation of bone with either Er:YAG or Er,Cr:YSGG lasers can be carried out to allow correct exposure of the fracture margin (Figs 30-35).

In the surgical adjunct to orthodontics, from gingival hyperplasia associated with orthodontic appliances, to the exposure of un-erupted teeth, the use of laser wavelengths can often enable simple procedures to be carried out without subjecting the child patient to additional anxiety[24-26] (Figs 36-39). Both short and long wavelengths can be used, taking care not to cause damage to the underlying tooth or bone, relative to wavelength. The control of bleeding will allow the placement of bonded brackets, without undue risk of failure.

SOFT TISSUES FIXED

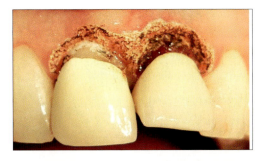
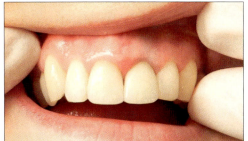

Fig. 12 (left) Immediately post-laser surgery

Fig. 13 (right) Final restorations at four weeks

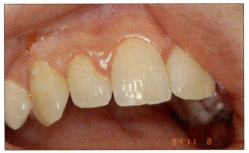
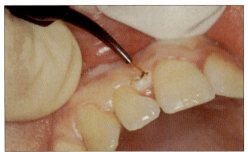

Fig. 14 (left) Inflammatory hyperplasia of UR 2 papilla

Fig. 15 (right) Nd:YAG laser fibre directed into discard; 100 mJ/20 pps/2.0 W

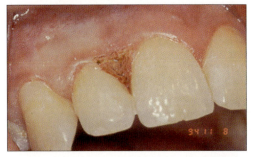
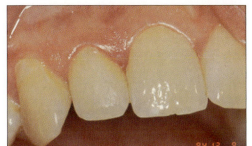

Fig. 16 (left) Immediately post-operative

Fig. 17 (right) Healing at one month

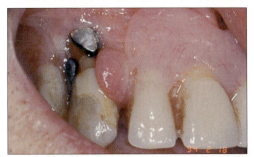
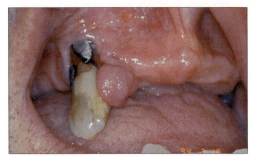

Fig. 18 (left) Irritation epulis associated with an ill-fitting denture flange

Fig. 19 (right) Pre-operative view

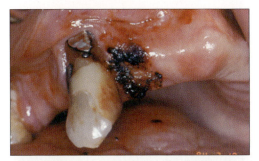
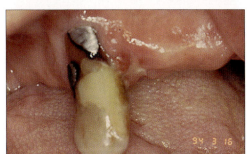

Fig. 20 (left) Nd:YAG laser excision

Fig. 21 (right) Healing at one month

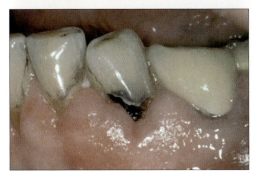
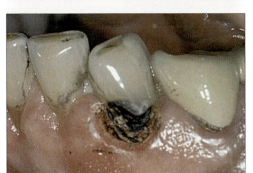

Fig. 22 (left) Gingival hyperplasia and associated cervical caries at LL 3

Fig. 23 (right) Soft tissue removed with CO_2 laser (1.5 W SP)

LASERS IN DENTISTRY

Fig. 24 (left) Cavity preparation completed with Er:YAG laser

Fig. 25 (right) Completed procedure

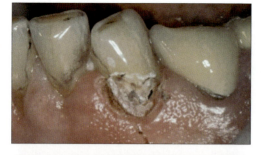
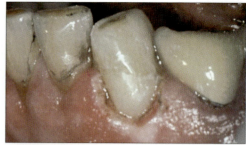

Fig. 26 (left) Buccal cusp UL4

Fig. 27 (right) Diode (810 nm) laser 2.0 W CW gingivectomy and pin placement

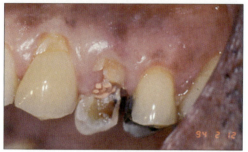
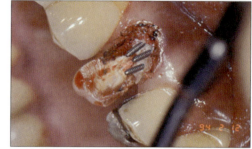

Fig. 28 (left) Crown fitted at three weeks

Fig. 29 (right) Follow-up at 10 years

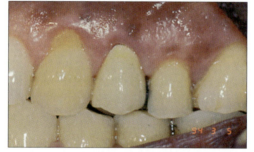
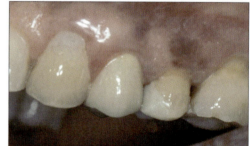

Fig. 30 (left) Fracture of palatal cusp UR 5

Fig. 31 (right) Following removal of tooth fragment, palatal soft tissue removed using CO_2 laser, 2.0 W SP

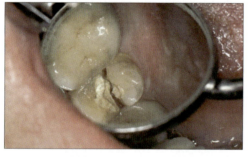
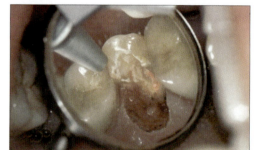

Fig. 32 (left) Bone removed using Er:YAG laser, 350 mJ/10 pps/3.5 W

Fig. 33 (right) Healing at two weeks. Tooth prepared for cast post and core

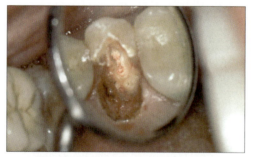
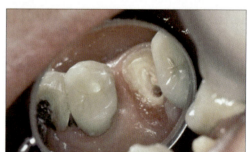

Fig. 34 (left) Healing at three weeks. Post and core cemented

Fig. 35 (right) Healing at four weeks. Final restoration

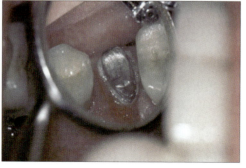
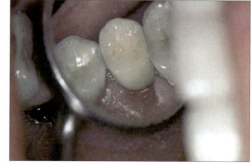

SOFT TISSUES FIXED

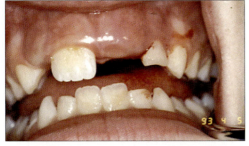
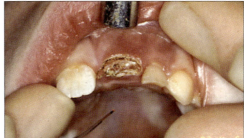
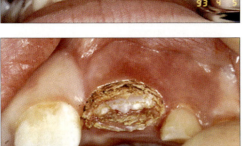
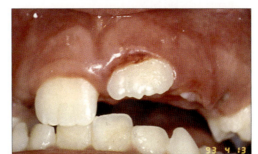
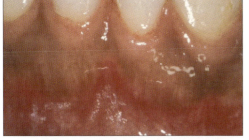
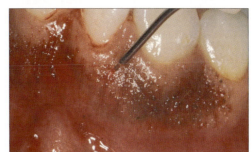
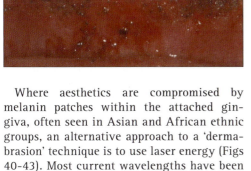
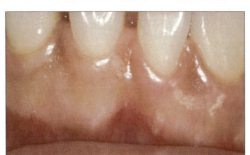

Fig. 36 (left) Unerupted UL 1 in an eight year-old patient

Fig. 37 (right) Use of Nd:YAG laser to expose tooth crown. 150 mJ/20 pps/3.0 W

Fig. 38 (left) Exposure complete. Note no damage to tooth crown

Fig. 39 (right) Spontaneous eruption and healing at one week

Fig. 40 (left) Melanin deposits

Fig. 41 (right) Selective absorption and ablation, using diode (810 nm) laser 1.4 W CW

Fig. 42 (left) Immediately post-operative

Fig. 43 (right) Healing at three weeks

Where aesthetics are compromised by melanin patches within the attached gingiva, often seen in Asian and African ethnic groups, an alternative approach to a 'dermabrasion' technique is to use laser energy (Figs 40-43). Most current wavelengths have been advocated, citing either selective pigment ablation with short wavelengths or superficial layer ablation of the tissue with longer wavelengths.[27-31] The correct use of the selected laser results in little or no discomfort or inflammation, compared to removal using rotary instrumentation.

CONCLUSION
The development of various laser systems in dentistry during the past 15 years has enabled a range of soft tissue procedures to be carried out. The benefits of haemostasis, sterility, reduced discomfort and obviation of dressings, merit advantages for both clinician and patient. The initial anecdotal reports of success that for many years sought to underline the credibility of laser use have been investigated through *in vitro* and *in vivo* studies. What is in little doubt is the predictability of laser use, based upon the biophysics of laser-tissue interaction; such an evidence-based approach continues to allow this treatment modality to expand its application in surgical dentistry.

1. Lanning S K, Waldrop T C, Gunsolley J C, Maynard J G. Surgical crown lengthening: evaluation of the biological width. *J Periodontol* 2003; **74:** 468-474.
2. Gracis S, Fradeani M, Celletti R, Bracchetti G. Biological integration of aesthetic restorations: factors influencing appearance and long-term success. *Periodontol 2000* 2001; **27:** 29-44.
3. Adams T C, Pang P K. Lasers in aesthetic dentistry. *Dent Clin North Am* 2004; **48:** 833-860, vi.
4. Kydd W L, Daly C H, Wheeler J B 3rd. The thickness measurements of masticatory mucosa in vivo. *Int Dent J* 1971; **21:** 430-441.
5. Pogrel M A, McCracken K J, Daniels T E. Histologic evaluation of the width of soft tissue necrosis adjacent to carbon dioxide laser incisions. *Oral Surg Oral Med Oral Pathol* 1990; **70:** 564-568.

6. Spencer P, Cobb C M, Wieliczka D M, Glaros A G, Morris P J. Change in temperature of subjacent bone during soft tissue laser ablation. *J Periodontol* 1998; **69:** 1278-1282.
7. Hall R R. The healing of tissues incised by a carbon dioxide laser. *Br J Surg* 1971; **58:** 222-225.
8. Fisher S E, Frame J W. The effects of the carbon dioxide surgical laser on oral tissues. *Br J Oral Maxillofac Surg* 1984; **22:** 414-425.
9. Pick R M, Pecaro B C. Use of the CO_2 laser in soft tissue dental surgery. *Lasers Surg Med* 1987; **7:** 207-213.
10. Wilder-Smith P, Arrastia A M, Schell M J, Grill G, Berns M W. Effect of Nd:YAG laser irradiation and root planning on the root surface: structural and thermal effects. *J Periodontol* 1995; **66:** 1032-1039.
11. White J M, Fagan M C, Goodis H E. Intra-pulpal temperatures during pulsed Nd:YAG laser treatment of dentin in vitro. *J Periodontol* 1994; **65:** 255-259.
12. Tokita Y, Sunakawa M, Suda H. Pulsed Nd:YAG laser irradiation of the tooth pulp in the cat: I. Effect of spot lasing. *Lasers Surg Med* 2000; **26:** 398-404.
13. Chaparro-Avendano A V, Berini-Aytes L, Gay-Escoda C. Peripheral giant cell granuloma. A report of five cases and review of the literature. *Med Oral Patol Oral Cir Bucal* 2005; **10:** 53-57; 48-52.
14. Wyman A, Duffy S, Sweetland H M, Sharp F, Rogers K. Preliminary evaluation of a new high power diode laser. *Lasers Surg Med* 1992; **12:** 506-509.
15. Hall R R, Hill D W, Beach A D. A carbon dioxide surgical laser. *Ann Royal Coll Surg Eng* 1971; **48:** 181-188.
16. Halldorsson T, Langerholc J. Thermodynamic analysis of laser irradiation of biological tissue. *Appl Opt* 1978; **17:** 3948-3958.
17. Goultschin J, Gazil D, Bichacho N, Bab I. Changes in teeth and gingiva of dogs following laser surgery: A block surface light microscope study. *Lasers Surg Med* 1988; **8:** 402-408.
18. Powell G L, Whisenant B K, Morton T H. Carbon dioxide laser oral safety parameters for teeth. *Lasers Surg Med* 1990; **10:** 389-392.
19. Barak S, Kaplan I. The CO_2 laser in the excision of gingival hyperplasia caused by nifedipine. *J Clin Periodontol* 1988; **15:** 633-635.
20. Roed-Petersen B. The potential use of CO_2-laser gingivectomy for phenytoin-induced gingival hyperplasia in mentally retarded patients. *J Clin Periodontol* 1993; **20:** 729-731.
21. Hylton R P. Use of CO_2 laser for gingivectomy in a patient with Sturge-Weber disease complicated by dilantin hyperplasia. *J Oral Maxillofac Surg* 1986; **44:** 646-648.
22. Rossmann J A, Ingles E, Brown R S. Multi-modal treatment of drug-induced gingival hyperplasia in a kidney transplant patient. *Compend Contin Educ Dent* 1994; **15:** 1266-1276.
23. Hattler A B, Kirschner R A, Susanin P B. Laser surgery for immunosuppressive gingival hyperplasia. *Periodontal Clin Investig* 1992; **14:** 18-20.
24. Parkins F M, Miller R L, Furnish G M, O'Toole T J. A preliminary report: YAG laser treatment in pediatric dentistry. *J Calif Dent Assoc* 1991; **19:** 43-44, 46-48, 50.
25. Convissar R A, Diamond L B, Fazekas C D. Laser treatment of orthodontically induced gingival hyperplasia. *Gen Dent* 1996; **44:** 47-51.
26. Sarver D M, Yanosky M. Principles of cosmetic dentistry in orthodontics: part 3. Laser treatments for tooth eruption and soft tissue problems. *Am J Orthod Dentofac Orthop* 2005; **127:** 262-264.
27. Esen E, Haytac M C, Oz I A, Erdogan O, Karsli E D. Gingival melanin pigmentation and its treatment with the CO_2 laser. *Oral Surg Oral Med Oral Pathol Oral Radiol Endod* 2004; **98:** 522-527.
28. Ishikawa I, Aoki A, Takasaki A A. Potential applications of Erbium:YAG laser in periodontics. *J Periodont Res* 2004; **39:** 275-285.
29. Tal H, Oegiesser D, Tal M. Gingival depigmentation by erbium:YAG laser: clinical observations and patient responses. *J Periodontol* 2003; **74:** 1660-1667.
30. Yousuf A, Hossain M, Nakamura Y, Yamada Y, Kinoshita J, Matsumoto K. Removal of gingival melanin pigmentation with the semiconductor diode laser: a case report. *J Clin Laser Med Surg* 2000; **18:** 263-266.
31. Atsawasuwan P, Greethong K, Nimmanon V. Treatment of gingival hyperpigmentation for esthetic purposes by Nd:YAG laser: report of 4 cases. *J Periodontol* 2000; **71:** 315-321.

IN BRIEF

- Laser use in periodontology includes the removal of intra-pocket diseased epithelium, bacterial and calculus accumulation and in the surgical correction of infra- and intra-bony pocketing.
- Laser use should be adjunctive to good periodontal therapy and not a replacement.
- Research into laser use in periodontology has been mixed. This may be due to the number of associated clinical parameters involved in *in vivo* investigations.
- All currently available laser wavelengths have been claimed to be effective in some or all aspects of the treatment of periodontal conditions. In addition, newer or experimental wavelengths may expand therapeutic use.
- Laser power levels must be kept to a minimum to avoid unwanted damage.

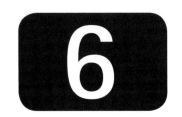

Lasers and soft tissue: periodontal therapy

Periodontology exists as a major specialty within clinical dentistry that has developed through the extensive research carried out into all parameters pertaining to a 'best practice' approach. With the advent of surgical lasers into clinical dentistry, considerable interest has been shown in the possible benefits that might be derived from the adjunctive effects of bacterial control and haemostasis that are associated with laser use. Despite the number of publications on the subject, there is still controversy over the use of lasers in periodontology. This chapter outlines the procedures that have been advocated for laser use and provides a review of the literature.

LASERS IN DENTISTRY

1. Introduction, history of lasers and laser light production
2. Laser-tissue interaction
3. Low-level laser use in dentistry
4. Lasers and soft tissue: 'loose' soft tissue surgery
5. Lasers and soft tissue: 'fixed' soft tissue surgery
6. **Lasers and soft tissue: periodontal therapy**
7. Surgical laser use in implantology and endodontics
8. Surgical lasers and hard dental tissue
9. Laser regulation and safety in general dental practice

SURGICAL LASERS AND PERIODONTOLOGY

The use of surgical lasers in periodontology is explored in three areas of treatment (Fig. 1):
- Removal of diseased pocket lining epithelium
- Bactericidal effect of lasers on pocket organisms
- Removal of calculus deposits and root surface detoxification.

Whatever benefits that may exist through the use of lasers, the prime responsibility of the clinician is to diagnose the existence of periodontal disease, establish and modify aggravating factors, treat the condition and seek to maintain health. As such, the use of lasers should be seen as adjunctive and supplemental to established protocols.

When integrated into a sound approach to pocket reduction, all current dental wavelengths have been advocated for the removal of diseased epithelium (Table 1). Added to the current wavelengths is the recent development of a frequency-doubled (wavelength-halved) Nd:YAG laser at 532 nm, termed the KTP laser, which has a range of action similar to that of the 810 nm diode. 'KTP' denotes potassium titanyl phosphate – the crystal used to effect the frequency doubling of the 1,064 nm wavelength.

The haemostatic advantage of using laser energy confers a controlling factor that is beneficial to both clinician and patient. Conceptually, in a periodontal pocket that is essentially supra-bony, the removal of hyperplastic soft tissue, together with a reduction in bacterial strains, renders the post-laser surgical site amenable to healing within normal limits. Where the pocket is infra-bony, a number of procedures have been advocated, including laser-ENAP[1] (excisional new attachment procedure), where the Nd:YAG (1,064 nm) laser is used in a non-flap procedure to reduce pocket depths of several millimetres, through a succession of treatment appointments.

A number of studies have been carried out to support the action of laser energy on various bacterial strains implicated in chronic periodontal disease. Short wavelength lasers interact with pigmented strains, whereas longer wavelength laser energy is absorbed by cellular water, leading to fragmentation of cellular structure.

Calculus, being a non-uniform mixture of inorganic salts, organic material, bacterial strains and water, can be viewed as a ready absorber of all wavelengths. However, the close association of calculus deposits with tooth and periodontal structures does pose a potential risk of collateral damage. Of the

LASERS IN DENTISTRY

Fig. 1 Areas of treatment where laser use has been demonstrated and investigated

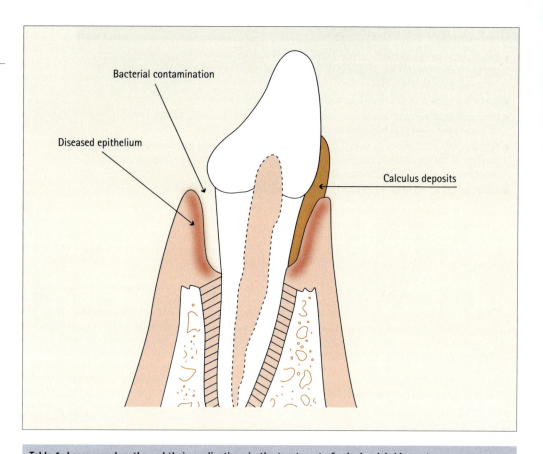

Table 1 Laser wavelengths and their applications in the treatment of sulcular debridement and removal/elimination of bacteria and calculus

Sulcular debridement	Bacteria	Calculus
Diode (810/980 nm)	Diode (810/980 nm)	Frequency-doubled alexandrite (377 nm)
Nd:YAG (1,064 nm)	Nd:YAG (1,064 nm)	-
Er,Cr:YSGG (2,780 nm)	Er,Cr:YSGG (2,780 nm)	Er,Cr:YSGG (2,780 nm)
Er:YAG (2,940 nm)	Er:YAG (2,940 nm)	Er:YAG (2,940 nm)
CO2 (10,600 nm)	CO2 (10,600 nm)	-

wavelengths investigated, erbium YAG (2,940 nm), erbium YSGG (2,780 nm) and frequency-doubled alexandrite (FDA, 377 nm) have been shown to interact and remove calculus selectively, with unwanted effects of a magnitude comparable with conventional techniques involving hand-instruments.

RISK ANALYSIS OF LASER USE

Notwithstanding non-structural factors such as local and systemic host susceptibility and genetic and lifestyle influences, the diseased periodontal pocket remains a complicated and potentially delicate structure to treat. Added to this, most laser delivery systems depend on an axial, end-on emission of light energy, which renders the target tissue liable to a potential build-up of direct and conductive heat effects. Consequently, there exists a profound need to limit laser power values to the minimum required to establish a desired effect and to avoid unwanted interaction, both with the tooth and periodontal attachment apparatus.

The lack of tactile feedback, together with the 'blind' treatment of non-reflected periodontal flaps, renders the need for caution as paramount. A detailed and thorough record of the diseased periodontium must be obtained prior to laser use as well as a respect for the need for conventional debridement to co-exist. In this way, only the proven benefits of laser use can be employed as an adjunctive, to maximise the outcome of the treatment in general. The temptation merely to expose a periodontal pocket to any laser energy, in the expectation that a magical resolution of the condition would ensue, undermines the professional approach to the patient and is to be deprecated.

DE-EPITHELIALISATION OF THE PERIODONTAL POCKET

The development of the quartz optic fibre delivery system associated with the diode and Nd:YAG group of lasers, with diameters of 200-320 µm, makes access into the periodontal pocket extremely easy. Longer wavelengths, where non-quartz deliveries are required, rely on fine bore waveguide probes and sapphire hand-piece tips, which are slightly wider, but which have been designed for the purpose (Figs 2-4).

Following the removal of all hard and soft deposits through scaling and/or root-planing, the pocket architecture is re-assessed, especially the depth. The laser probe or fibre is measured to a distance of one to two millimetres short of the pocket depth and is inserted at an angle to maintain contact with the soft tissue wall at all times. Using laser power values sufficient to ablate the epithelial lining (approximately 0.8 W CW diode, 100 mJ/20 pps, 2.0 W Nd:YAG and Er:YAG/YSGG, 1.0 W CW CO_2), the laser probe is used in a light contact, sweeping mode to cover the entire soft tissue lining. Ablation should commence near the base of the pocket and proceed upwards, by slowly removing the probe (Fig. 5).

It is often seen that some bleeding of the pocket site will occur. This may be due to disruption of the fragile inflamed pocket epithelium, but in terms of laser haemostasis, the power levels employed are low and designed to remove the epithelial surface and decontaminate. Regular inspection should be carried out to prevent the build-up of ablation debris on the fibre or probe end, which should be cleaned with damp sterile gauze. Each pocket site should be treated for 20-30 seconds, amounting possibly to two minutes per tooth site, with re-treatment at approximate weekly intervals during any maximum four-week period. Gentle pocket probing and measurement to establish benefits of treatment should be resisted during this period.

Several laser-related studies have appeared in the periodontal literature to date.[2-14] Case reports have recommended the diode laser (810 nm), along with the Nd:YAG (1,064 nm), for treatment of periodontal pockets by laser sub-gingival curettage. However, these reports offer no evidence that these procedures are superior to conventional scaling and root planing alone. The American Academy of Periodontology, in its position statement on lasers in ENAP,[15] states *'The Academy is not aware of any published data that indicates that the ENAP laser procedure is any more effective for these purposes than traditional scaling and planing'*.[12,16-22] This is sharply contrasted by reports by Gregg and McCarthy, reported in later journals.[23-25] In 2004 in a study presented by Evans[26] to review the new attachment procedure on a sample of six cases, evidence was given to show new cementum and bone growth, including periodontal ligament. What must be considered is the extent to which such treatment can be empirically assessed, when many deep periodontal lesions often merit tooth stabilisation and occlusal guarding. Furthermore, there are limited evidence-based clinical trials to substantiate the clinical benefits of laser-assisted sub-gingival curettage and the presence of root surface damage following this procedure has been reported.[27] The carbon dioxide laser has been shown to enhance periodontal therapy through a de-epithelial technique in conjunction with traditional flap surgery procedures. It has been demonstrated that the CO_2 laser can be used to de-epithelialise the flap during surgery and it has enhanced reduction in periodontal probing depths.[4,13,14] Several controlled studies have assessed the use of laser therapy combined with conventional scaling and root planing, although these investigations demonstrated no benefit or only slightly improved treatment outcomes.[28-31]

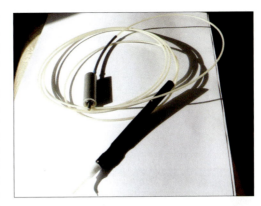

Fig. 2 Quartz fibre assembly for use with eg diode and Nd:YAG lasers

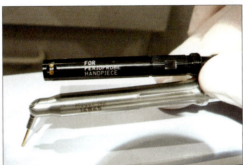

Fig. 3 Focussed waveguide tip for use with CO_2 laser wavelength

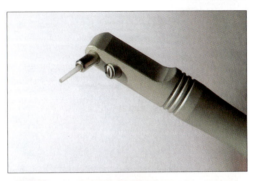

Fig. 4 Sapphire tip for use with Er:YAG laser wavelength

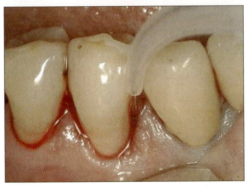

Fig. 5 Quartz fibre (diode laser) being used in a periodontal pocket. Some bleeding is expected, as sufficient laser energy is used only to remove the epithelial lining of the pocket

LASERS IN DENTISTRY

Fig. 6 (left) Angled tip for use with Er:YAG laser in calculus removal

Fig. 7 (right) Quartz tip for use with frequency-doubled alexandrite laser (377 nm)

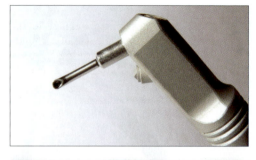
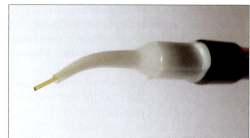

Fig. 8 (left) Radiograph of infra-bony pocket associated with LL first molar

Fig. 9 (right) Mucogingival flap raised to show granulation tissue within pocket

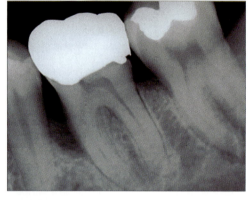
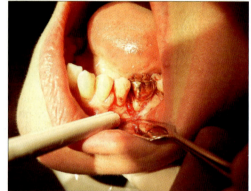

Fig. 10 (left) Subgingival calculus deposits being removed from infra-bony pocket with Er:YAG laser

Fig. 11 (right) Defect filled with allograft bone matrix

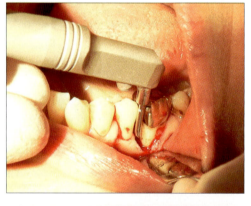
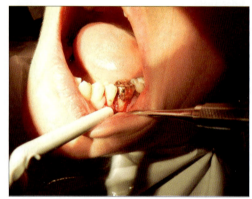

Fig. 12 (left) Healing site at three months

Fig. 13 (right) Radiograph showing bony infill of defect

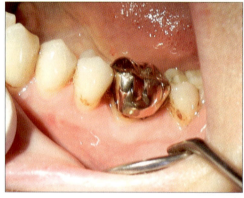
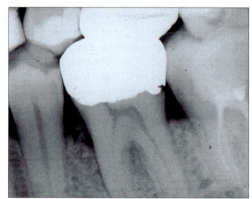

Fig. 14 (left) Pre-operative crown lengthening site (reproduced with permission of Dr Donald Coluzzi, Redwood City, CA, USA)

Fig. 15 (right) Flap raised, showing level of alveolar bone (reproduced with permission of Dr Donald Coluzzi, Redwood City, CA, USA)

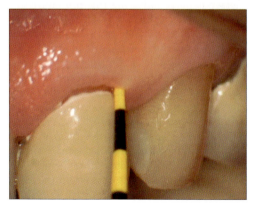
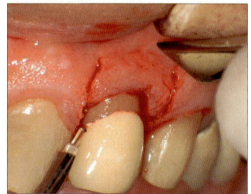

PERIODONTAL

Conversely, a study in 2003 by Schwarz et al.[32] using an erbium laser indicated that non-surgical periodontal therapy with both an Er:YAG laser plus scaling/root planing (SRP) and an Er:YAG laser alone, led to significant improvements in all clinical parameters investigated; also, the combined treatment Er:YAG laser plus SRP did not seem to additionally improve the outcome of the therapy compared to Er:YAG laser alone.

LASER BACTERIAL REDUCTION

Among the bacteria most implicated in periodontal disease and bone loss are *Actinobacillus actinomycetemcomitans, Porphyromonas gingivalis* and *Bacteroides forsythus*. Other bacteria associated with periodontal disease are *Treponema denticola, T. sokranskii* and *Prevotella intermedia*. These latter bacteria, together with *P. gingivalis*, are frequently present at the same sites and are associated with deep periodontal pockets. Most studies reported in the literature focus on the *in vitro* action of various laser wavelengths on these selected bacterial species.

The effectiveness of any laser wavelength is dependant upon the absorption characteristics of the target bacterial structure (water, pigment) being matched by the incident beam. In addition, *in vivo*, the indeterminate existence of definable parameters of laser energy dosage, concentration of bacterial colonies and accuracy of exposure, may give rise to some scepticism as to the predictability of this therapy. However, the conjunctive use of lasers within conventional periodontal therapy, both *in vitro* and *in vivo*, does support the clinical picture of a beneficial role of lasers in pocket decontamination.

Many studies have been carried out to demonstrate the effectiveness of laser energy on bacterial strains found in the diseased pocket.[33-36] Some studies have reported on the additional role of laser use in conjunction with scaling and root planing and locally-applied antibiotic preparations.[37,38] It is evident from the numerous studies undertaken in this field that the levels of incident energy employed are essentially sufficient to ablate bacterial cellular structure; what appears to be difficult to quantify is the protocol required to render any periodontal pocket 'sterile'.

A recent study by Bornstein[39] cites an innovative use of a diode (810-830 nm) laser, in conjunction with methylene blue, to address some of the difficulties of using this wavelength within the confines of the periodontal pocket. All too often, the build-up of char and de-natured protein material on the delivery fibre of the (emitting CW) diode laser, results in the development of a carbonised tip, with the temperature rising in excess of 700°C. If not removed, this leads to an attenuation of the subsequent laser beam, replaced by the secondary emission of radiant thermal energy from the carbonised deposits ('hot-tip effect'). The conductive heat effects that result lead to unwanted damage to the delicate tissue structure. The use of a chemical mediator, such as methylene blue, serves to act as a heat sink for the thermal energy and to enhance bacteriocidal action. This proposal, along with extension of the concept of photo-activated disinfection in cavity preparation, remains the subject of further investigation.

LASERS AND CALCULUS REMOVAL

The predominance of Nd:YAG and CO_2 laser wavelengths in dentistry until 1994 gave good ground to the viewpoint that calculus removal using laser energy was either incomplete or fraught with damage potential to surrounding tissues.[23,40-42] The development of Er:YAG and Er,Cr:YSGG, together with innovative near-UV wavelengths such as frequency-doubled alexandrite (FDA, 377 nm), has given encouragement to the safe use of these lasers in calculus removal.

In order to provide access to calculus deposits, specific laser hand-piece tips have been developed for use with the mid-infrared erbium wavelengths (Fig. 6).

The shorter FDA wavelength is delivered through an optic fibre (Fig. 7) and to date, remains a developmental machine. However, further investigation is anticipated into the use of diode-based lasers of wavelengths in the region of 400 nm, which would still prove interactive with calculus, but avoid some claims that the 377 nm wavelength might give rise to ionising effects in target tissue.

The poorly-calcified deposits, together with higher water content, has rendered supra- and sub-gingival calculus susceptible to de-fragmentation through photo-mechanical ablation with the erbium group.[43-45] Potentially, this enables deposits to be removed using laser energy levels less than those required for ablation of dental hard tissue (Figs 8-13). This is borne out in a study by Aoki *et al.*,[46] where laser power levels as low as 0.3 Watts have been shown to be sufficient to ablate calculus. Intriguingly, the same centre reported that the efficiency of Er:YAG in calculus removal was less than that of ultrasonic instrumentation.[47]

The advantage of using the 377 nm laser is based on studies that have shown the differential increased absorption of this laser by calculus, as opposed to cementum and dentine.[48-50]

In addition to the treatment of periodontal disease, erbium YAG and erbium YSGG lasers can be used to carry out bone remodelling. Whilst the effectiveness of these wavelengths on bone is discussed in greater detail in the later chapter on lasers and hard tissue, the clinical results obtained within the management of the alveolus/periodontium complex are most promising (Figs 14-18).

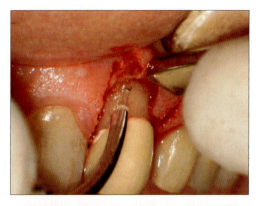

Fig. 16 Erbium YAG laser being used with water spray to remove unwanted bone. Note the angulation of tip to avoid damage to the root surface (reproduced with permission of Dr Donald Coluzzi, Redwood City, CA, USA)

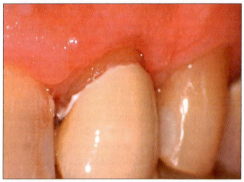

Fig. 17 Healed surgical site at one month (reproduced with permission of Dr Donald Coluzzi, Redwood City, CA, USA)

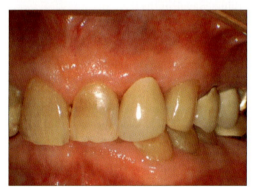

Fig. 18 Final restoration in place (reproduced with permission of Dr Donald Coluzzi, Redwood City, CA, USA)

CONCLUSION

Considerable debate continues as to the effectiveness and/or efficiency of lasers in the field of periodontology. In those geographical areas of the world where hygienists and other auxiliaries are able to carry out surgical pocket debridement, there is considerable enthusiasm for use. Generally, conventional opinion remains unequivocal as to laser usage, despite the number of studies carried out. The many anecdotal reports as to beneficial use of lasers serve only to establish an opinion as to laser effectiveness and certainly there is agreement amongst protagonists as to the improvement in tissue health following laser treatment. The difficulties in establishing a series of protocols, addressing differences in periodontal pocket architecture, presence and extent of disease and deposits, laser power parameters and which laser wavelength is at all superior, will only serve to allow the debate to continue. What is quite evident is that, whilst any 'closed' procedure within the pocket demands skill and consideration, the use of any laser should be adjunctive and thorough knowledge of potential damaging factors appreciated.

Perhaps nowhere else is the maxim 'minimal power to achieve the desired effect' more appropriate that in this field of dentistry. From the review of the literature, it is personally felt that there is a need for greater control of studies that reflect objectivity and reduce subjectivity, in order to provide confidence for practitioners in maximising the benefits of lasers. Through this approach, laser use can be anticipated to gain greater acceptance in the field of periodontology.

Permission granted by Dr Donald Coluzzi, Redwood City, California, USA to reproduce his clinical photographs of crown lengthening treatment is acknowledged.

1. Millennium Dental Technologies, Inc. *Dent Prod Rep* 1999; **33:** 40.
2. Spencer P, Cobb C M, Wieliczka D M, Glaros A G, Morris P J. Change in temperature of subjacent bone during soft tissue laser ablation. *J Periodontol* 1998; **69:** 1278-1282.
3. Fujii T, Baehni P C, Kawai O, Kwawkami T, Matsuda K, Kowashi Y. Scanning electron microscopic study of the effects of Er:YAG laser on root cementum. *J Periodontol* 1998; **69:** 1283-1290.
4. Rossmann J A, Cobb C M. Lasers in periodontal therapy. *Periodontol 2000* 1995; **9:** 150-164.
5. Israel M, Rossmann J A, Froum S J. Use of the carbon dioxide laser in retarding epithelial migration: a pilot histological human study utilizing case reports. *J Periodontol* 1995; **66:** 197-204.
6. Williams T M, Cobb C M, Rapley J W, Killoy W J. Histologic evaluation of alveolar bone following CO_2 laser removal of connective tissue from periodontal defects. *Int J Periodontics Restorative Dent* 1995; **15:** 497-506.
7. Wilder-Smith P, Arrastia A A, Schell M J, Liaw L H, Grill G, Berns M W. Effect of Nd:YAG laser irradiation and root planing on the root surface: structural and thermal effects. *J Periodontol* 1995; **66:** 1032-1039.
8. Rizoiu I M, Eversole L R, Kimmel A I. Effects of an erbium, chromium:yttrium, scandium, gallium garnet laser on mucocutaneous soft tissues. *Oral Surg Oral Med Oral Pathol* 1996; **82:** 386-395.
9. Yamaguchi H, Kobayashi K, Reiko O *et al*. Effects of irradiation of an erbium:YAG laser on root surfaces. *J Periodontol* 1997; **68:** 1151-1155.
10. Israel M, Cobb C M, Rossmann J A, Spencer P. The effects of the CO_2, Nd:YAG and Er:YAG lasers with and without surface coolant on the tooth root surfaces: an in vitro study. *J Clin Periodontol* 1997; **24:** 595-602.
11. Krause L S, Cobb C M, Rapley J W, Killoy W J, Spencer P. Laser irradiation of bone: I. An in vitro study concerning the effects of the CO_2 laser on oral mucosa and subjacent bone. *J Periodontol* 1997; **68:** 872-880.
12. Gopin B W, Cobb C M, Rapley J W, Killoy W J. Histologic evaluation of soft tissue attachment to CO_2 laser treated root surfaces: an in vivo study. *Int J Periodontics Restorative Dent* 1997; **17:** 317-325.
13. Centty I G, Blank L W, Levy B A *et al*. Carbon dioxide laser for de-epithelialization of periodontal flaps. *J Periodontol* 1997; **68:** 763-769.
14. Israel M, Rossmann J A. An epithelial exclusion technique using the CO_2 laser for the treatment of periodontal defects. *Compend Contin Educ Dent* 1998; **19:** 1238-1245.
15. American Academy of Periodontology. *Statement regarding use of dental lasers for excisional new attachment procedure (ENAP)*. Chicago: AAP, 1999.
16. Trylovich D J, Cobb C M, Pippin D J, Spencer P, Killoy W J. The effects of the Nd:YAG laser on in vitro fibroblast attachment to endotoxin-treated root surfaces. *J Periodontol* 1992; **63:** 626-632.
17. Morlock B J, Pippin D J, Cobb C M, Killoy W J, Rapley J W. The effect of Nd:YAG laser exposure on root surfaces when used as an adjunct to root planing. *J Periodontol* 1992; **63:** 637-641.
18. Spencer P, Trylovich D J, Cobb C M. Photoacoustic FTIR spectroscopy of lased cementum surfaces. *J Periodontol* 1992; **63:** 633-636.
19. Spencer P, Cobb C M, McCollum M H, Wieliczka D M. The effects of CO_2 laser and Nd:YAG with and without water/air surface cooling on tooth root structure: correlation between FTIR spectroscopy and histology. *J Periodont Res*

1996; **31:** 453-462.
20. Thomas D, Rapley J W, Cobb C M, Spencer P, Killoy W J. Effects of the Nd:YAG laser and combined treatments on in vitro fibroblast attachment to root surfaces. *J Clin Periodontol* 1994; **21:** 38-44.
21. Cobb C M, Spencer P, McCollum M H. Histologic comparison of the CO_2 and Nd:YAG lasers with and without water/air surface cooling on tooth root structure. *Proc SPIE* 1995; **2394:** 20-31.
22. Radvar M, Creanor S L, Gilmour W H et al. An evaluation of the effects of an Nd:YAG laser on subgingival calculus, dentine and cementum. An in vitro study. *J Clin Periodontol* 1995; **22:** 71-77.
23. Gregg R H, McCarthy D K. Laser ENAP for periodontal bone regeneration. *Dent Today* 1998; **17(5):** 88-91.
24. Gregg R H, McCarthy D K. Laser ENAP for periodontal ligament regeneration. *Dent Today* 1998; **17(11):** 86-89.
25. Gregg R H, McCarthy D K. Laser economics: periodontal therapy. *Dent Econ* 1998; **88:** 42-44.
26. Yukna R A, Evans G, Vastardis S, Carr R L. Human periodontal regeneration following laser assisted new attachment procedure. *Proc IADR/AADR/CADR* 82nd General Session. Hawaii, 2004.
27. Cobb C M, McCawley T K, Killoy W J. A preliminary study on the effects of the Nd:YAG laser on root surfaces and subgingival microflora in vivo. *J Periodontol* 1992; **63:** 701-707.
28. Yilmaz S, Kuru L, Noyan U, Argun D, Kadir T. Effect of gallium arsenide diode laser on human periodontal disease: a microbiological and clinical study. *Lasers Surg Med* 2002; **30:** 60-66.
29. Liu C M, Hou L T, Wong M Y, Lan W H. Comparison of Nd:YAG laser versus scaling and root planing in periodontal therapy. *J Periodontol* 1999; **70:** 1276-1282.
30. Schwarz F, Sculean A, Georg T, Reich E. Periodontal treatment with an Er:YAG laser compared to scaling and root planning. A controlled clinical study. *J Periodontol* 2001; **72:** 361-367.
31. Neill M E, Mellonig J T. Clinical efficacy of the Nd:YAG laser for combination periodontitis therapy. *Pract Periodontics Aesthet Dent* 1997; **9:** 1-5.
32. Schwarz F, Sculean A, Berakdar M, Georg T, Reich E, Becker J. Clinical evaluation of an Er:YAG laser combined with scaling and root planing for non-surgical periodontal treatment. A controlled, prospective clinical study. *J Clin Periodontol* 2003; **30:** 26-34.
33. Harris D M, Yessik M. NdYAG better than diode. *Lasers Surg Med* 2004; **35:** 206-213.
34. Grassi R F, Pappalardo S, Frateiacci A et al. Antibacterial effect of Nd:YAG laser in periodontal pockets decontamination: an in vivo study. *Minerva Stomatol* 2004; **53:** 355-359 [article in Italian].
35. Moritz A, Schoop U, Goharkhay K et al. Treatment of periodontal pockets with a diode laser. *Lasers Surg Med* 1998; **22:** 302-311.
36. Coffelt D W, Cobb C M, MacNeill S, Rapley J W, Killoy W J. Determination of energy density threshold for laser ablation of bacteria. An in vitro study. *J Clin Periodontol* 1997; **24:** 1-7.
37. Miyazaki A, Yamaguchi T, Nishikata J et al. Effects of Nd:YAG and CO_2 laser treatment and ultrasonic scaling on periodontal pockets of chronic periodontitis patients. *J Periodontol* 2003; **74:** 175-180.
38. Noguchi T, Sanaoka A, Fukuda M, Suzuki S, Aoki T. Combined effects of Nd:YAG laser irradiation with local antibiotic application into periodontal pockets. *J Int Acad Periodontol* 2005; **7:** 8-15.
39. Bornstein E. Method and dosimetry for thermolysis and removal of biofilm in the periodontal pocket with near-infrared diode lasers: a case report. *Dent Today* 2005; **24(4):** 60, 62, 64-70.
40. Arcoria C J, Vitasek-Arcoria B A. The effects of low-level energy density Nd:YAG irradiation on calculus removal. *J Clin Laser Med Surg* 1992; **10:** 343-347.
41. Cobb C M. Lasers in periodontics: use and abuse. *Compend Contin Educ Dent* 1997; **18:** 847-852, 854-855, 858-859.
42. Tucker D, Cobb C M, Rapley J W, Killoy W J. Morphologic changes following in vitro CO_2 laser treatment of calculus-ladened root surfaces. *Lasers Surg Med* 1996; **18:** 150-156.
43. Folwaczny M, Mehl A, Haffner C, Benz C, Hickel R. Root substance removal with Er:YAG laser radiation at different parameters using a new delivery system. *J Periodontol* 2000; **71:** 147-155.
44. Frentzen M, Braun A, Aniol D. Er:YAG laser scaling of diseased root surfaces. *J Periodontol* 2002; **73:** 524-530.
45. Eberhard J, Ehlers H, Falk W, Acil Y, Albers H K, Jepsen S. Efficacy of subgingival calculus removal with Er:YAG laser compared to mechanical debridement: an in situ study. *J Clin Periodontol* 2003; **30:** 511-518.
46. Aoki A, Ando Y, Watanabe H, Ishikawa I. In vitro studies on laser scaling of subgingival calculus with an erbium:YAG laser. *J Periodontol* 1994; **65:** 1097-1106.
47. Aoki A, Miura M, Akiyama F et al. In vitro evaluation of Er:YAG laser scaling of subgingival calculus in comparison with ultrasonic scaling. *J Periodont Res* 2000; **35:** 266-277.
48. Pilgrim C, Rechmann P, Goldin D, Hennig T. Measurement of efficiency in calculus removal with a frequency-doubled alexandrite laser on pigs' jaws. *Proc SPIE* 2000; **3910:** 50-58.
49. Rechmann P, Hennig T, Reichart P. Periodontal treatment with the frequency-doubled alexandrite laser in dogs. *Proc SPIE* 2000; **3910:** 35-41.
50. Rechmann P, Hennig T, Hamid M, Sadegh M, Goldin D. Light and scanning electron microscope investigations comparing calculus removal using an Er:YAG laser and a frequency-doubled alexandrite laser. *Proc SPIE* 1997; **2973:** 53-59.

IN BRIEF

- Laser use in implantology has been historically controversial.
- The development of a range of laser wavelengths has shown the adjunctive use of lasers to be more beneficial, both in the healthy and diseased implant case.
- Laser use in endodontics has advocated benefits in all stages of treatment. However, some are based on anecdote or innovation.
- The greater investigation into all wavelengths has centred on the anti-bacterial action of laser light energy.

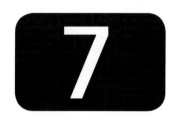

Surgical laser use in implantology and endodontics

The use of surgical lasers has been advocated to aid in the placement and second stage recovery of dental implants, together with soft tissue contouring. In addition, laser use has been suggested as an aid in decontamination of the implant surface in cases of peri-implantitis. In endodontics, the association of laser energy with dentine hypersensitivity, bacteriocidal action and pulp-capping, has led to a growing number of reports as to its beneficial use, together with claims of morphological changes in the canal wall, to enhance endodontic treatment success.

LASERS IN DENTISTRY

1. Introduction, history of lasers and laser light production
2. Laser-tissue interaction
3. Low-level laser use in dentistry
4. Lasers and soft tissue: 'loose' soft tissue surgery
5. Lasers and soft tissue: 'fixed' soft tissue surgery
6. Lasers and soft tissue: periodontal therapy
7. **Surgical laser use in implantology and endodontics**
8. Surgical lasers and hard dental tissue
9. Laser regulation and safety in general dental practice

THE USE OF LASERS IN IMPLANTOLOGY

Surgical lasers can be used in a variety of ways with regard to implantology, ranging from placement, second stage recovery and gingival management, through to the treatment of peri-implantitis. Within this range of usage, dependant on wavelength employed, exists the ablation of target tissue and the ability to reduce bacterial contamination.

Whilst there is a general acceptance that lasers are capable of accurate cutting of materials and tissue, there is no evidence-based advocacy as to the use of any laser wavelength in producing a fully-prepared osteotomy site for the placement of root-form dental implants. However, there are anecdotal reports of the use of erbium YAG and erbium YSGG lasers to establish a controlled incision of overlying gingival tissue and to initiate a breach of the cortical bone plate, prior to the use of conventional implant drills. Such techniques, although intrinsically correctly based on predictable laser-tissue interaction, run the risk of scepticism amongst practitioners more allied to a conventional surgical approach to implant placement.

The fundamental controversy?
With all other predisposing factors addressed, the fundamental key to success in implant placement is the apposition of normal healing bone onto the implant surface. The preparation of the osteotomy site demands a technique whereby the local temperature does not exceed 47°C.[1] Inasmuch as the prime interaction in laser use results in the conversion of incident electromagnetic energy into heat energy, any therapeutic use of lasers in implant dentistry must address this fact. Added to this, once in place, the possibility of implant surface damage arising from incident laser light must be avoided.

The first dental laser, the Nd:YAG (1,064 nm) offered advantages of soft tissue ablation, haemostasis and bacterial control. However, the free-running pulsed emission mode can give rise to peak power values per pulse of >1,000 Watts. Research into the use of this laser as an adjunctive to implantology, drew conclusions that the penetrating and high peak heat energy effects produced during soft tissue and peri-implant treatment, caused damage to both the implant surface and surrounding bone.[2-4] This led to a general deprecation of laser use in connection with implants, which remained for several years.

With the further development of other laser wavelengths, investigations were carried out to establish whether these newer lasers

IMPLANTS/ENDO

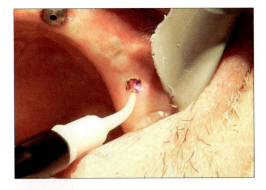
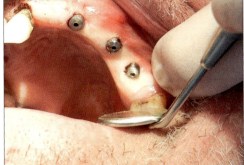

Fig. 1 (left) Implant cover screw access obtained using diode (810 nm) laser

Fig. 2 (right) Healing cap in place

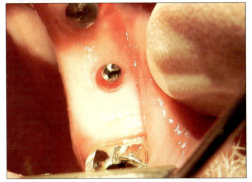
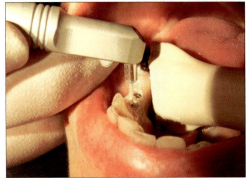

Fig. 3 (left) Soft tissue healing at 10 days

Fig. 4 (right) Implants uncovered using Er:YAG (2,940 nm) laser without water spray

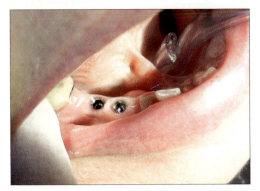
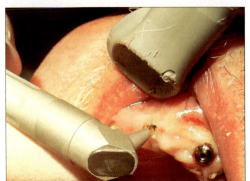

Fig. 5 (left) Healing at one week

Fig. 6 (right) Second stage recovery using CO_2 laser (10,600 nm)

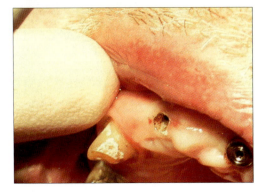
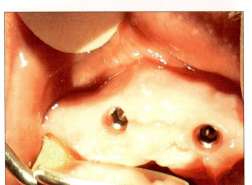

Fig. 7 (left) Laser use complete

Fig. 8 (right) Healing at 10 days

would cause damage. The general parameters would include the emission mode of the laser (continuous wave (CW), gated pulsed (GP) or free-running pulsed (FRP)), the nature of the target tissue and type of laser-tissue interaction. Other investigations centred around the material used in implant manufacture, its reflectivity, whether the titanium was coated and, generally, the conductive effects of heat through the implant into surrounding bone. Of prime concern is the potential damage to the implant surface and the escalation of heat effects beyond the 47°C threshold in adjacent bone.

Titanium as a metal exhibits reflectivity to incident light energy. With regard to the wavelengths of current lasers, the reflectivity is lowest in the range 780-900 nm, rising as the wavelength increases towards 10,600 nm (CO_2 laser emission).[5] This would suggest that shorter wavelengths are most damaging, as the low reflectivity would allow greater heat effects to build up, and is in keeping with studies carried out with the Nd:YAG laser. However, there is evidence to suggest that the diode wavelength group, delivered in low power CW values (1-2 Watts average power), cause minimal damage to the implant[2] or

Fig. 9 Two implants uncovered with scalpel-assisted flap. Poor tissue contour due to early loss of sutures

Fig. 10 Excess soft tissue being removed using CO_2 (10,600 nm) laser. Note use of damp gauze to prevent distant damage

Fig. 11 Immediate post-laser exposure of healing caps and re-contouring of soft tissue outline

Fig. 12 Soft tissue healing at two weeks

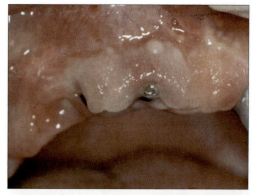

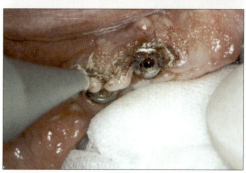

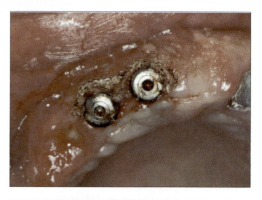

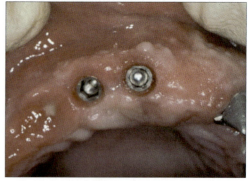

surrounding bone.[6,7] This is explained by the fact that the Nd:YAG, Er,Cr:YSGG and Er:YAG emission modes (FRP), result in high peak power values and heat production (>several hundred °C). Despite the damaging effects of carbon dioxide laser light on bone, several studies have borne out the high reflectivity of titanium to this wavelength, in reporting low thermal effects on the metal surface[8-15] and non-damaging effects on the metal composition.[16]

Soft tissue management associated with implants
Based on laser-tissue interaction characteristics, all laser wavelengths are suitable for the second stage recovery of implants, provided care is exercised to avoid contact with the implant body (Figs 1-8). The ablation of soft tissue leads to precise and predictable healing and often this procedure can be carried out using topical anaesthesia.

Suggested energy levels of one to two Watts (CW diode), 150 mJ/15 pps (Nd:YAG), 200-250 mJ/10 pps (erbium group) and one to two Watts (CO_2), appear to be appropriate in removing gingival tissue overlying the implant cover screw. The prime advantages of laser use in this procedure would be haemostasis, facilitating easier visual access to the cover screw, production of a protective coagulum as an aid to healing and patient comfort during and after treatment.

Minor surgical correction of the gingival margin can be carried out, to assist adequate implant exposure or to establish the correct emergence profile of the trans-mucosal element (Figs 9-19).

As with gingivoplasty around natural teeth, a near-excision approach can be adopted with final detachment of the discard with a sharp curette; alternatively, laboratory-made acrylic copings can be fitted.

Laser use in peri-implantitis
As with conventional treatment approaches, assessment must be made as to the causative factors associated with the condition (infection, occlusion, implant overloading and other local, systemic and life-style factors), and whether the implant is essentially saveable.

Peri-implantitis is recognised as a rapidly progressive failure of osseo-integration,[17] in which the production of bacterial toxins precipitates inflammatory change and bone loss.[18] The development of peri-implantitis is not restricted to any one type of implant design or construction[19,20] and is cited as one of the greater causes of implant loss.[21,22] Inasmuch as mechanical debridement together with chemical decontamination (eg chlorhexidine digluconate, citric acid) of the exposed implant surface, with or without site-specific antibiotics, has proved somewhat effective, the possibility to remove bacterial colonisation with an appropriate laser wavelength might well be seen as an added benefit.[23-32]

In spite of the risks inherent in using a microsecond pulsed laser, studies by Kreisler *et al.*, using an Er:YAG laser (60-120 mJ/10 pps – 0.6-1.2 W), and Miller, using an Er,Cr:YSGG laser with similar energy parameters, found bacterial kills >99%, without reported damaging effects on the implant surface.[33,34]

Meticulous attention must be given to curettage of granulation tissue; a laser wavelength that is non-injurious to bone (eg erbium group plus water) can be used to remove this tissue, although careful use of a diode laser, avoiding heat effects (a water spray can be used) and restricting its use to fragmentation and

IMPLANTS/ENDO

Table 1 Laser wavelengths and their possible application in endodontics	
Laser	Procedure
Diode (810-980 nm)	Desensitisation, pulp capping, root canal disinfection
Nd:YAG (1,064 nm)	Desensitisation, pulp capping, pulpectomy, root canal cleaning and disinfection
Er,Cr:YSGG (2,780 nm)	Access cavity preparation, root canal shaping, cleaning and disinfection
Er:YAG (2,940 nm)	Access cavity preparation, pulpectomy, root canal shaping, cleaning and disinfection
CO_2 (10,600 nm)	Desensitisation, pulp capping, pulpectomy

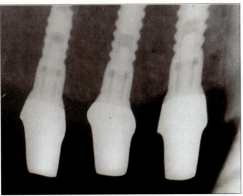

Fig. 13 Transmucosal elements in place at three implant sites in the UR posterior region

ablation, can be employed. The ability of laser energy in bacterial decontamination appears to place its use above that of other modalities (Figs 20-23).

However, there is less evidence of beneficial use where the implant is coated with a ceramic or hydroxyapatite; this may be mostly due to the micro-complex surface irregularities, which have been shown to harbour bacteria and foreign ions in a failing situation.[35,36]

LASERS AND ENDODONTICS

All current dental laser wavelengths have been used in a wide range of endodontic treatments, either to aid the preparation stages or obturation techniques of root canal therapy or to alleviate low-grade pulpal injury.[37,38]

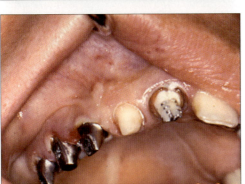

Fig. 14 Diode (810 nm) laser used to contour soft tissue around TMEs

The areas of endodontics where laser use has been investigated include the following:
- Direct pulp capping
- Removal of pulpal tissue
- Access/shaping of canal walls and morphological changes in structure
- Bacterial decontamination
- Sealing with or removal of gutta percha obturation material
- Root dentine (cervical) desensitisation.

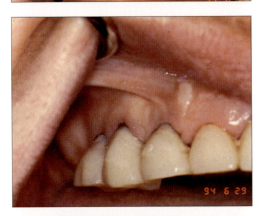

Fig. 15 Immediately post-laser surgery with provisional crowns in place

As with laser use in the debridement of the periodontal pocket, it should be remembered that non-visual access places a potential limit on the control exercised by the operator in using laser energy within the root canal. In addition, laser use should be adjunctive to good clinical practice if benefits are to be maximised. Wherever laser use is indicated, it is recommended that this should be evidence-based and, if deemed appropriate, complementary to all other treatment measures that might be considered. Table 1 lists the procedures that have been advocated and investigated in the field of endodontics and the current commercially available laser wavelengths that are applicable.

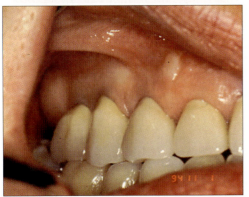

Fig. 16 Finished result at five months

Pulp capping and pulpotomy

The consideration for pulp capping and/or pulpotomy using a laser should complement contemporary protocols for such action. Vital pulp exposure (arising from caries or trauma) and subsequent local action, leading to preservation of vital tissue, is contentious in the permanent dentition and success rates are low. It is suggested that permanent teeth

LASERS IN DENTISTRY

with open apices or deciduous teeth offer better chances of pulp reparation.[39,40] However, the use of laser energy to aid haemostasis and remove bacterial contamination in order that a reparative dentine bridge could form can offer increased chances of a successful resolution.[41-43]

In a study of 83 patients with 93 teeth treated through a pulp capping procedure, Santucci reported survival rates over 54 months of 43% in teeth treated with calcium hydroxide/resin cement, as opposed to 90% in those teeth treated with Nd:YAG laser and a similar capping cement.[44] Moritz et al. (260 teeth treated, 130 study/130 control), reported a tooth vitality two-year survival rate of 93% (control 66%), using a super-pulsed CO_2 laser under similar conditions.[45]

Laser technique involving the exposed vital pulp should be carried out under rubber dam, to prevent contamination with salivary bacteria. Minimal energy levels (1-2 W average power) per wavelength should be employed to provide haemostasis and sterilise the cut surface. A calcium hydroxide dressing should be applied directly, prior to completion of cavity restoration.

Access/shaping of canal walls and morphological changes in structure

The accepted interaction of the Er:YAG and Er,Cr:YSGG lasers with dental hard tissue makes these wavelengths ideal for removal of dentine overlying the pulp chamber.[46] The benefit of non-tactile stimulation can aid this procedure in teeth that are tender to percussion and where anaesthesia is incomplete or insufficient.

Within the confines of the root canal, the use of laser wavelengths without water cooling can lead to a potential high rise in temperature. Risks associated include melting/cracking of dentine walls and trans-apical irradiation of the tooth socket.[47] With short infrared and CO_2 lasers, if benefit is to be obtained, power levels of 0.75-1.5 W should be considered maximal. With water-assisted erbium lasers, power values of 150-250 mJ/4-8 pps are considered suitable, but it is essential to allow water to reach the ablation site, in order to prevent over-heating and cavitation of canal walls.[48-50]

In order to address the end-on emission of laser light from the delivery system, modified intra-canal instruments have been developed[51,52] and pre-trial experimental devices to produce non-axial laser light propagation along optic fibres have been investigated (Figs 24-26).

With mechanical canal preparation, a smear layer is often produced, which can harbour bacteria. Most laser wavelengths will remove the smear layer and can be used in conjunction with irrigants and chelating agents such as NaOCl or EDTA. The Nd:YAG laser has been extensively investigated, but many reports have been made regarding melting and carbonisation.[53-56] It is considered that the erbium group of laser wavelengths is best placed to achieve this, without causing damaging temperature rise.[57]

Bacterial decontamination

Peri-radicular lesions are diseases either primarily or secondarily caused by micro-organisms. Conventional treatments suggest the combination of mechanical debridement and chemical anti-bacterial agents.[58,59]

As discussed previously, the anti-bacterial action of laser light is a major benefit of this treatment modality, although in complex canal systems, the use of NaOCl or H_2O_2 has been shown to be more effective.[60-62] The fine (200-320 µm) diameters of quartz optic fibres associated with diode and Nd:YAG lasers has enabled these wavelengths to be easily used in bacterial decontamination of the root canal (Figs 27-35).[63-65]

Of the current lasers available, the CO_2 wavelength would appear least

Fig. 17 Laboratory made acrylic copings fitted to implant abutments to aid in protecting implant neck from thermal energy. Nd:YAG (1,064 nm) laser

Fig. 18 Immediately post-laser surgery

Fig. 19 Peri-implant soft tissue contour at one month

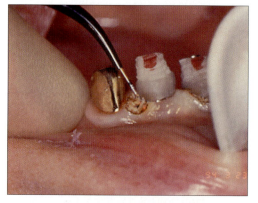

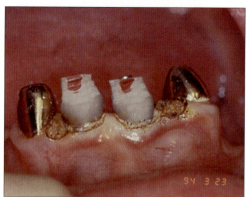

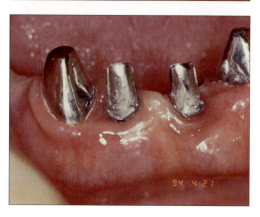

IMPLANTS/ENDO

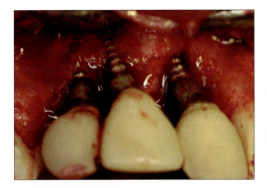

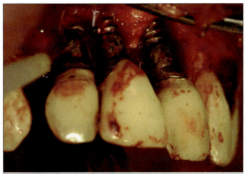

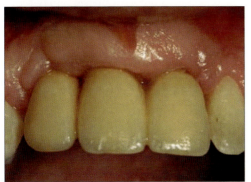

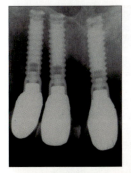 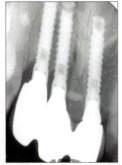

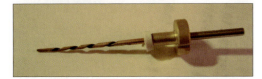

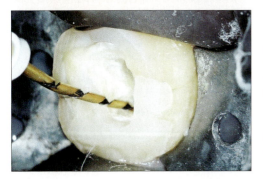

Fig. 20 Peri-implantitis resulting in labial and interstitial bone loss in 21/1 region (figure courtesy of Professor G. Romanos, New York University, New York, USA)

Fig. 21 (right) Following removal of granulation tissue, diode (810 nm) laser used to remove bacteria from implant surfaces (figure courtesy of Professor G. Romanos, New York University, New York, USA)

Fig. 22 Post-surgery healing at three months, with new coronal restorations (figure courtesy of Professor G. Romanos, New York University, New York, USA)

Fig. 23 Pre-surgery (left) and three months (right) radiographs, following open flap debridement and bone grafting (figure courtesy of Professor G. Romanos, New York University, New York, USA)

Fig. 24 Endodontic laser tip for use with Er:YAG laser

Fig. 25 Laser tip being used in root canal. Laser energy is reflected off inclined surfaces and through gaps in spiral to exit at 90° to the axis

successful in effecting bacterial decontamination[66] and the effectiveness of laser use appears to depend on fluence values and direct access.[67] In addition, some concern has been expressed that the plume produced during laser action might allow bacterial contamination to spread.[68,69] As with laser bacterial action in other clinical sites, sub-ablative energy levels should be employed for all wavelengths.

Comparative studies on two common bacterial pathogens, *Escherichia coli* and *E. faecalis* have shown that the more complex cell wall of the latter can reduce the effectiveness of laser action. One study by Schoop et al. concluded that diode 810 nm and erbium YAG were better placed to ablate significant numbers of *E. faecalis* organisms.[70] Curiously, in another study by Jha investigating the Er,Cr:YSGG laser, no beneficial bacteriocidal effect could be demonstrated, with either lasers or rotary instrumentation.[71] As was reported in the paper on LLLT (*BDJ* 2007; 202: 131-138), some studies have been carried out, both *in vitro* and *in vivo*, into the use of photo-activated disinfection in eliminating intra-canal pathogenic species.[72-74] In common with studies on many areas of bacterial populations in dentistry, inclusion/exclusion criteria remain significant in determining outcome and can make direct comparison difficult.

Sealing with or removal of gutta percha obturation material

A number of studies have been carried out to establish the usefulness of lasers in the softening and obturation of gutta percha in the root canal (Fig. 36).[75-79] However, the development of thermoplastic materials and instruments for such purposes has rendered such application comparatively time consuming and expensive.[47]

Dentine hypersensitivity

In the absence of any other aetiological factors, 'true' dentine hypersensitivity can be due to gingival recession or toothbrush abrasion and may cause pulpal stimulation through dynamic changes in the intra-tubular proteinaceous fluid.[80] Laser-mediated treatment of exposed dentine has been either to address the patency of tubular openings, causing closure of tubule openings to a depth of several microns, or to coagulate the tubular contents.[81-83] Kimura, in a review of the literature from 1985-2000, ranged the effectiveness of lasers in the treatment of dentine hypersensitivity from 5-100%, dependant upon wavelength and fluence.[84] The most commonly explored lasers are the low-level diode (HeNe 633 nm, GaAlAs 810 nm) group and moderate power diode and Nd:YAG.[85-90] Of these, the use of the Nd:YAG wavelength

LASERS IN DENTISTRY

Fig. 26 (left) 'Micro-probe' insert for use with CO_2 laser

Fig. 27 (right) 320 µm diameter quartz fibre for use with diode (810–980 nm) and Nd:YAG (1,064 nm) lasers. A canula is usually fitted onto the fibre. Size comparable with #30 endodontic file. Fibre length can be measured in the same way as hand files

Fig. 28 (left) Fibre with HeNe aiming beam being introduced into extracted root canal

Fig. 29 (right) Optic fibre inserted to two millimetres short of working length. Note 'fluorescence' effect of light through tubular dentine. Invisible laser light is thought to behave in a similar manner

Fig. 30 (left) 200 µm diameter fibre in clinical use in endodontics

Fig. 31 (right) Measurement of fibre length

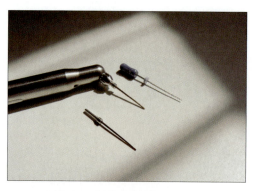
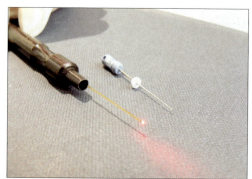
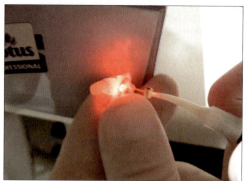
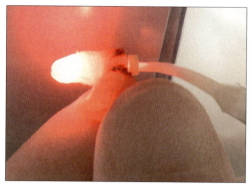
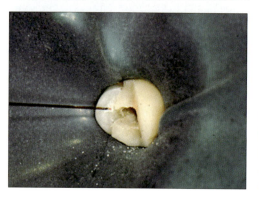
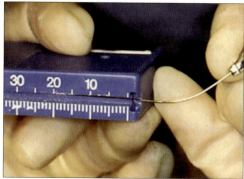
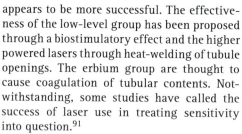

appears to be more successful. The effectiveness of the low-level group has been proposed through a biostimulatory effect and the higher powered lasers through heat-welding of tubule openings. The erbium group are thought to cause coagulation of tubular contents. Notwithstanding, some studies have called the success of laser use in treating sensitivity into question.[91]

Energy levels when using hard lasers must be sufficiently low in order to avoid pulpal damage (shorter wavelengths), or tissue ablation (longer wavelengths) and should be of an order of 0.3–0.5 W average power.

CONCLUSION

The use of lasers in implantology and endodontics has prompted controversy, due either to the essential photothermal action of high powered lasers and its potential for collateral thermal damage, or to the risks associated with 'blind' techniques. The considerable number of investigations carried out into the many permutations of laser wavelengths and target sites has allowed a refinement of criteria and a balanced approach to the claimed success, or otherwise, of laser use. Anecdotal claims as to the effectiveness of this modality continue to drive the need for critical evaluation.

Permission granted by Professor G. Romanos, New York University, New York, USA to reproduce his clinical photographs of peri-implantitis treatment is acknowledged.

1. Eriksson A, Albrektsson T. Temperature threshold levels for heat-induced bone tissue injury. A vital microscoping study in the rabbit. *J Prosthet Dent* 1983; **50:** 101–107.
2. Romanos G E, Everts H, Nentwig G H. Effects of diode and Nd:YAG laser irradiation on titanium discs: a scanning electron microscope examination. *J Periodontol* 2000; **71:** 810–815.
3. Block C, Mayo J, Evans G. Effects of the Nd:YAG dental laser on plasma-sprayed and hydroxyapatite coated titanium dental implants: surface alterations and attempted sterilization. *Int J Oral Maxillofac Implants* 1992; **7:** 441–449.
4. Kreisler M, Götz H, Duschner H, d'Hoedt B. Effect of the Nd:YAG, Ho:YAG, Er:YAG, CO_2 and GaAlAs laser irradiation on surface properties of endosseous dental implants. *Med Laser Appl* 2001; **16:** 152.
5. Rechmann P, Sadegh H, Goldin D, Hennig T. Surface morphology of implants after laser irradiation. *Dtsch Zahnärztl Z* 2000; **55:** 371–376 [in German].
6. Kreisler M, Al Haj H, d'Hoedt B. Temperature changes induced by 809-nm GaAlAs laser at the implant-bone interface during simulated surface decontamination. *Clin Oral Implants Res* 2003; **14:** 91–96.
7. Kreisler M, Schoof J, Langnau E, Al Haj H, d'Hoedt B. Temperature elevations in endosseous dental implants and

IMPLANTS/ENDO

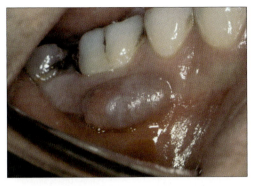

Fig. 32 Buccal swelling associated with acute periapical abscess, LR 6

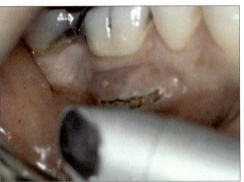

Fig. 33 'No touch' incision of swelling using CO_2 (10,600 nm) laser

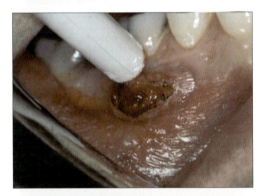

Fig. 34 Aspiration of pus. Note absence of bleeding along incision line

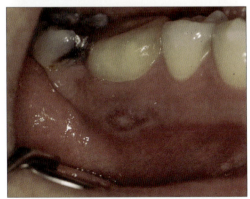

Fig. 35 Lesion at two weeks, following root canal therapy

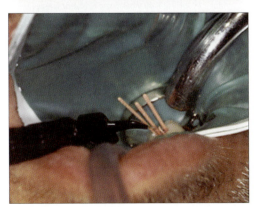

Fig. 36 Nd:YAG laser being used to section gutta percha points

the peri-implant bone during diode-laser-assisted surface decontamination. *Proc SPIE* 2002; **4610:** 21-30.
8. Deppe H, Greim H, Brill T, Wagenpfeil S. Titanium deposition after peri-implant care with the carbon dioxide laser. *Int J Oral Maxillofac Implants* 2002; **17:** 707-714.
9. Swift J, Jenny J, Hargreaves K. Heat generation in hydroxyapatite-coated implants as a result of CO_2 laser application. *Oral Surg Oral Med Oral Pathol Oral Radiol Endod* 1995; **79:** 410-415.
10. Oyster D, Parker W, Gher M. CO_2 lasers and temperature changes of titanium implants. *J Periodontol* 1995; **66:** 1017-1024.
11. Ganz C. Evaluation of the safety of the carbon dioxide laser used in conjunction with root form implants. A pilot study. *J Prosthet Dent* 1994; **71:** 27-30.
12. Barak S, Horowitz I, Katz J, Oelgiesser D. Thermal changes in endosseous root-form implants as a result of CO_2 laser application: an in vitro and in vivo study. *Int J Oral Maxillofac Implants* 1998; **13:** 666-671.
13. Shibli J, Theodoro L, Haypek P, Garcia V, Marcantonio E. The effect of CO_2 laser irradiation on failed implant surfaces. *Implant Dent* 2004; **13:** 342-351.
14. Mouhyi J, Sennerby L, Nammour S, Guillaume P, Van Reck J. Temperature increases during surface decontamination of titanium implants using CO_2 laser. *Clin Oral Implant Res* 1999; **10:** 54-61.
15. Wooten C, Sullivan S, Surpure S. Heat generation by superpulsed CO_2 lasers on plasma-sprayed titanium implants: an in vitro study. *Oral Surg Oral Med Oral Pathol Oral Radiol Endod* 1999; **88:** 544-548.
16. Mouhyi J, Sennerby L, Wennerberg A, Louette P, Dourov N, van Reck J. Re-establishment of the atomic composition and the oxide structure of contaminated titanium surfaces by means of carbon dioxide laser and hydrogen peroxide: an in vitro study. *Clin Implant Dent Relat Res* 2000; **2:** 190-202.
17. Mombelli A. Etiology, diagnosis, and treatment considerations in peri-implantitis. *Curr Opin Periodontol* 1997; **4:** 127-136.
18. Leonhardt A, Renvert S, Dahlen G. Microbial findings at failing implants. *Clin Oral Implants Res* 1999; **10:** 339-345.
19. Martins M C, Abi-Rached R S, Shibli J A, Araujo M W, Marcantonio E Jr. Experimental peri-implant tissue breakdown around different dental implant surfaces: clinical and radiographic evaluation in dogs. *Int J Oral Maxillofac Implants* 2004; **19:** 839-848.
20. Shibli J A, Martins M C, Lotufo R F, Marcantonio E Jr. Microbiologic and radiographic analysis of ligature-induced peri-implantitis with different dental implant surfaces. *Int J Oral Maxillofac Implants* 2003; **18:** 383-390.
21. Kourtis S G, Sotiriadou S, Voliotis S, Challas A. Private practice results of dental implants. Part I: survival and evaluation of risk factors – Part II: surgical and prosthetic complications. *Implant Dent* 2004; **13:** 373-385.
22. Oh T J, Yoon J, Misch C E, Wang H L. The causes of early implant bone loss: myth or science? *J Periodontol* 2002; **73:** 322-333.
23. Romeo E, Ghisolfi M, Murgolo N, Chiapasco M, Lops D, Vogel G. Therapy of peri-implantitis with resective surgery. A 3-year clinical trial on rough screw-shaped oral implants. Part I: clinical outcome. *Clin Oral Implants Res* 2005; **16:** 9-18.
24. Augthun M, Tinschert J, Huber A. In vitro studies on the effect of cleaning methods on different implant surfaces. *J Periodontol* 1998; **69:** 857-864.
25. Buchter A, Meyer U, Kruse-Losler B, Joos U, Kleinheinz J. Sustained release of doxycycline for the treatment of peri-implantitis: randomised controlled trial. *Br J Oral Maxillofac Surg* 2004; **42:** 439-444.
26. Klinge B, Gustafsson A, Berglundh T. A systematic review of the effect of anti-infective therapy in the treatment of peri-implantitis. *J Clin Periodontol* 2002; **29 (Suppl 3):** 213-225.
27. Tang Z, Cao C, Sha Y, Lin Y, Wang X. Effects of non-surgical treatment modalities on peri-implantitis. *Zhonghua Kou Qiang Yi Xue Za Zhi* 2002; **37:** 173-175.
28. Bunetel L, Guerin J, Agnani G *et al.* In vitro study of the effect of titanium on Porphyromonas gingivalis in the presence of metronidazole and spiramycin. *Biomaterials* 2001; **22:** 3067-3072.
29. Leonhardt A, Dahlen G, Renvert S. Five-year clinical, microbiological, and radiological outcome following treatment of peri-implantitis in man. *J Periodontol* 2003; **74:** 1415-1422.

30. Walsh L. The use of lasers in implantology: an overview. *J Oral Implantol* 1992; **18:** 335-340.
31. Haas R, Dörtbudak O, Mensdorff-Pouilly N, Mailath G. Elimination of bacteria on different implant surfaces through photosensitization and soft laser. *Clin Oral Implants Res* 1997; **8:** 249-254.
32. Kato T, Kusakari H, Hoshino E. Bactericidal efficacy of carbon dioxide laser against bacteria-contaminated implants and subsequent cellular adhesion to irradiated area. *Lasers Surg Med* 1998; **23:** 299-309.
33. Kreisler M, Kohnen W, Marinello C et al. Bactericidal effect of the Er:YAG laser on dental implant surfaces: an in vitro study. *J Periodontol* 2002; **73:** 1292-1298.
34. Miller R J. Treatment of the contaminated implant surface using the Er,Cr:YSGG laser. *Implant Dent* 2004; **13:** 165-170.
35. Ichikawa T, Hirota K, Kanitani H, Miyake Y, Matsumoto N. In vitro adherence of Streptococcus constellatus to dense hydroxyapatite and titanium. *J Oral Rehabil* 1998; **25:** 125-127.
36. MacDonald D E, Betts F, Doty S B, Boskey A L. A methodological study for the analysis of apatite-coated dental implants retrieved from humans. *Ann Periodontol* 2000; **5:** 175-184.
37. Stabholz A, Sahar-Helft S, Moshonov J. Lasers in endodontics. *Dent Clin North Am* 2004; **48:** 809-832.
38. Kimura Y, Wilder-Smith P, Matsumoto K. Lasers in endodontics: a review. *Int Endod J* 2000; **33:** 173-185.
39. Shoji S, Nakamura M, Horiuchi H. Histopathological changes in dental pulps irradiated by CO_2 laser: a preliminary report on laser pulpotomy. *J Endod* 1985; **11:** 773-780.
40. Dang J, Wilder-Smith P, Peavy G. Clinical preconditions and treatment modality: effects on pulp surgery outcome. *Lasers Surg Med* 1998; **22:** 25-29.
41. Liu H, Yan M M, Zhao E Y, Chen L, Liu H W. Preliminary report on the effect of Nd: YAG laser irradiation on canine tooth pulps. *Chin J Dent Res* 2000; **3(4):** 63-65.
42. Jayawardena J A, Kato J, Moriya K, Takagi Y. Pulpal response to exposure with Er:YAG laser. *Oral Surg Oral Med Oral Pathol Oral Radiol Endod* 2001; **91:** 222-229.
43. Kimura Y, Yonaga K, Yokoyama K, Watanabe H, Wang X, Matsumoto K. Histopathological changes in dental pulp irradiated by Er:YAG laser: a preliminary report on laser pulpotomy. *J Clin Laser Med Surg* 2003; **21:** 345-350.
44. Santucci P J. Dycal versus Nd:YAG laser and Vitrebond for direct pulp capping in permanent teeth. *J Clin Laser Med Surg* 1999; **17:** 69-75.
45. Moritz A, Schoop U, Goharkhay K, Sperr W. Advantages of a pulsed CO_2 laser in direct pulp capping: a long-term in vivo study. *Lasers Surg Med* 1998; **22:** 288-293.
46. Chen W H. Laser root canal therapy. *J Indiana Dent Assoc* 2002-2003; **81:** 20-23.
47. Anic I, Tachibana H, Matsumoto K, Qi P. Permeability, morphologic and temperature changes of canal dentine walls induced by Nd:YAG, CO_2 and argon lasers. *Int Endod J* 1996; **29:** 13-22.
48. Ebihara A, Majaron B, Liaw L H, Krasieva T B, Wilder-Smith P. Er:YAG laser modification of root canal dentine: influence of pulse duration, repetitive irradiation and water spray. *Lasers Med Sci* 2002; **17:** 198-207.
49. Yamazaki R, Goya C, Yu D G, Kimura Y, Matsumoto K. Effects of erbium,chromium:YSGG laser irradiation on root canal walls: a scanning electron microscopic and thermographic study. *J Endod* 2001; **27:** 9-12.
50. Kimura Y, Yonaga K, Yokoyama K, Kinoshita J, Ogata Y, Matsumoto K. Root surface temperature increase during Er:YAG laser irradiation of root canals. *J Endod* 2002; **28:** 76-78.
51. Shoji S, Hariu H, Horiuchi H. Canal enlargement by Er:YAG laser using a cone-shaped irradiation tip. *J Endod* 2000; **26:** 454-458.
52. Kesler G, Gal R, Kesler A, Koren R. Histological and scanning electron microscope examination of root canal after preparation with Er:YAG laser microprobe: a preliminary in vitro study. *J Clin Laser Med Surg* 2002; **20:** 269-277.
53. Kaitsas V, Signore A, Fonzi L, Benedicenti S, Barone M. Effects of Nd: YAG laser irradiation on the root canal wall dentin of human teeth: a SEM study. *Bull Group Int Rech Sci Stomatol Odontol* 2001; **43:** 87-92.
54. Levy G. Cleaning and shaping the root canal with a Nd:YAG laser beam: a comparative study. *J Endod* 1992; **18:** 123-127.
55. Miserendino L, Levy G, Rizoiu I. Effects of Nd:YAG laser on the permeability of root canal wall dentin. *J Endod* 1995; **21:** 83-87.
56. Zhang C, Kimura Y, Matsumoto K, Harashima T, Zhou H. Effects of pulsed Nd:YAG laser irradiation on root canal wall dentin with different laser initiators. *J Endod* 1998; **24:** 352-355.
57. Matsuoka E, Kimura Y, Matsumoto K. Studies on the removal of debris near the apical seats by Er:YAG and assessment with a fiberscope. *J Clin Laser Med Surg* 1998; **16:** 255-261.
58. Siqueira Junior J F. Strategies to treat infected root canals. *J Calif Dent Assoc* 2001; **29:** 825-837.
59. Piccolomini R, D'Arcangelo C, D'Ercole S, Catamo G, Schiaffino G, De Fazio P. Bacteriologic evaluation of the effect of Nd:YAG laser irradiation in experimental infected root canals. *J Endod* 2002; **28:** 276-278.
60. Schoop U, Moritz A, Kluger W et al. The Er:YAG laser in endodontics: results of an in vitro study. *Lasers Surg Med* 2002; **30:** 360-364.
61. Perin F M, Franca S C, Silva-Sousa Y T et al. Evaluation of the antimicrobial effect of Er:YAG laser irradiation versus 1% sodium hypochlorite irrigation for root canal disinfection. *Aust Endod J* 2004; **30:** 20-22.
62. Folwaczny M, Mehl A, Jordan C, Hickel R. Antibacterial effects of pulsed Nd:YAG laser radiation at different energy settings in root canals. *J Endod* 2002; **28:** 24-29.
63. Rooney J, Midda M, Leeming J. A laboratory investigation of the bactericidal effect of a Nd:YAG laser. *Br Dent J* 1994; **176:** 61-64.
64. Fegan S, Steiman H. Comparative evaluation of the antibacterial effects of intracanal Nd:YAG laser irradiation: an in vitro study. *J Endod* 1995; **21:** 415-417.
65. Moritz A, Gutknecht N, Gohrakhay K, Schoop U, Wernisch J, Sperr W. In vitro irradiation of infected root canals with a diode laser: results of microbiologic, infrared spectrometric, and stain penetration examinations. *Quintessence Int* 1997; **28:** 205-209.
66. Le Goff A, Dautel-Morazin A, Guigand M, Vulcain J M, Bonnaure-Mallet M. An evaluation of the CO_2 laser for endodontic disinfection. *J Endod* 1999; **25:** 105-108.
67. Kreisler M, Kohnen W, Beck M et al. Efficacy of NaOCl/H_2O_2 irrigation and GaAlAs laser in decontamination of root canals in vitro. *Lasers Surg Med* 2003; **32:** 189-196.
68. McKinley I, Ludlow M. Hazards of laser smoke during endodontic therapy. *J Endod* 1994; **20:** 558-559.
69. Hardee M, Miserendino L, Kos W, Walia H. Evaluation of the antibacterial effects of intracanal Nd:YAG laser irradiation. *J Endod* 1994; **20:** 377-380.
70. Schoop U, Kluger W, Moritz A, Nedjelik N, Georgopoulos A, Sperr W. Bactericidal effect of different laser systems in the deep layers of dentin. *Lasers Surg Med* 2004; **35:** 111-116.
71. Jha D, Guerrero A, Ngo T, Helfer A, Hasselgren G. Inability of laser and rotary instrumentation to eliminate root canal infection. *J Am Dent Assoc* 2006; **137:** 67-70.
72. Williams J A, Pearson G J, John Colles M. Antibacterial action of photoactivated disinfection {PAD} used on endodontic bacteria in planktonic suspension and in artificial and human root canals. *J Dent* 2006; **34:** 363-371.
73. Bonsor S J, Nichol R, Reid T M S, Pearson G J. Microbiological evaluation of photo-activated disinfection in endodontics (an in vivo study). *Br Dent J* 2006; **200:** 337-341.
74. Lee M T, Bird P S, Walsh L J. Photo-activated disinfection of root canals: a new role for lasers in endodontics. *Aust Endod J* 2004; **30:** 93-98.
75. Anjo T, Ebihara A, Takeda A, Takashina M, Sunakawa M, Suda H. Removal of two types of root canal filling material using pulsed Nd:YAG laser irradiation. *Photomed Laser Surg* 2004; **22:** 470-476.
76. Viducic D, Jukis S, Karlovic Z, Bozic Z, Miletic I, Anic I. Removal of gutta-percha from root canals using an Nd: YAG laser. *Int Endod J* 2003; **36:** 670-673.
77. Carvalho C A, Valera M C, Gown-Soares S, de Paula Eduardo C. Effects of Nd:YAG and Er:YAG lasers on the sealing of root canal fillings. *J Clin Laser Med Surg* 2002; **20:** 215-219.
78. Maden M, Gorgul G, Tinaz A C. Evaluation of apical leakage of root canals obturated with Nd: YAG laser-softened gutta-percha, System-B, and lateral condensation techniques. *J Contemp Dent Pract* 2002; **3:** 16-26.
79. Kimura Y, Yonaga K, Yokoyama K, Matsuoka E, Sakai K, Matsumoto K. Apical leakage of obturated canals prepared by Er:YAG laser. *J Endod* 2001; **27:** 567-570.
80. Absi E G, Addy M, Adams D. Dentine hypersensitivity. A study of the patency of dentinal tubules in sensitive and non-sensitive cervical dentine. *J Clin Periodontol* 1987; **14:** 280-284.

81. Liu H C, Lin C P, Lan W H. Sealing depth of Nd:YAG laser on human dentinal tubules. *J Endod* 1997; **23:** 691-693.
82. Schwarz F, Arweiler N, Georg T, Reich E. Desensitizing effects of an Er:YAG laser on hypersensitive dentine. *J Clin Periodontol* 2002; **29:** 211-215.
83. Zhang C, Matsumoto K, Kimura Y, Harashima T, Takeda F H, Zhou H. Effects of CO_2 laser in treatment of cervical dentinal hypersensitivity. *J Endod* 1998; **24:** 595-597.
84. Kimura Y, Wilder-Smith P, Yonaga K, Matsumoto K. Treatment of dentine hypersensitivity by lasers: a review. *J Clin Periodontol* 2000; **27:** 715-721.
85. Marsilio A L, Rodrigues J R, Borges A B. Effect of the clinical application of the GaAlAs laser in the treatment of dentine hypersensitivity. *J Clin Laser Med Surg* 2003; **21:** 291-296.
86. Corona S A, Nascimento T N, Catirse A B, Lizarelli R F, Dinelli W, Palma-Dibb R G. Clinical evaluation of low-level laser therapy and fluoride varnish for treating cervical dentinal hypersensitivity. *J Oral Rehabil* 2003; **30:** 1183-1189.
87. Walsh L J. The current status of low level laser therapy in dentistry. Part 2. Hard tissue applications. *Aust Dent J* 1997; **42:** 302-306.
88. Renton-Harper P, Midda M. Nd:YAG laser treatment of dentinal hypersensitivity. *Br Dent J* 1992; **172:** 13-16.
89. Lan W H, Lee B S, Liu H C, Lin C P. Morphologic study of Nd:YAG laser usage in treatment of dentinal hypersensitivity. *J Endod* 2004; **30:** 131-134.
90. Ciaramicoli M T, Carvalho R C, Eduardo C P. Treatment of cervical dentin hypersensitivity using neodymium: yttrium-aluminum-garnet laser. Clinical evaluation. *Lasers Surg Med* 2003; **33:** 358-362.
91. Lier B B, Rosing C K, Aass A M, Gjermo P. Treatment of dentin hypersensitivity by Nd:YAG laser. *J Clin Periodontol* 2002; **29:** 501-506.

IN BRIEF

- Lasers have been advocated to address the clinical preparation of restorative cavities and also the pain associated with conservative dentistry.
- All oral hard tissues can be ablated with laser energy.
- Precision, preservation of healthy tissue and control of temperature rise are hallmarks of correct laser use on hard tissue.
- The development of interceptive techniques to address early carious lesions may herald a more widespread use of lasers in restorative dentistry.

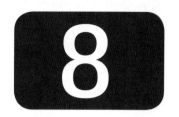

Surgical lasers and hard dental tissue

The cutting of dental hard tissue during restorative procedures presents considerable demands on the ability to selectively remove diseased carious tissue, obtain outline and retention form and maintain the integrity of supporting tooth tissue without structural weakening. In addition, the requirement to preserve healthy tissue and prevent further breakdown of the restoration places the choice of instrumentation and clinical technique as prime factors for the dental surgeon. The quest for an alternative treatment modality to the conventional dental turbine has been, essentially, patient-driven and has led to the development of various mechanical and chemical devices. The review of the literature has endorsed the beneficial effects of current laser machines. However utopian, there is additional evidence to support the development of ultra-short (nano- and femto-second) pulsed lasers that are stable in use and commercially viable, to deliver more efficient hard tissue ablation with less risk of collateral thermal damage. This chapter explores the interaction of laser energy with dental hard tissues and bone and the integration of current laser wavelengths into restorative and surgical dentistry.

LASERS IN DENTISTRY

1. Introduction, history of lasers and laser light production
2. Laser-tissue interaction
3. Low-level laser use in dentistry
4. Lasers and soft tissue: 'loose' soft tissue surgery
5. Lasers and soft tissue: 'fixed' soft tissue surgery
6. Lasers and soft tissue: periodontal therapy
7. Surgical laser use in implantology and endodontics
8. **Surgical lasers and hard dental tissue**
9. Laser regulation and safety in general dental practice

THE DEVELOPMENT OF THE 'LASER DRILL'

The fundamental concept of laser energy with oral tissue components has been explored in earlier chapters in this book. The first laser wavelengths to be made available for general dental practice use were the Nd:YAG (1,064 nm) laser together with the carbon dioxide (10,600 nm) laser, which had already found acceptance in oral and maxillofacial surgery. Both laser wavelengths, in their emission mode configuration, had been in use for some time in their capacity to ablate soft tissue. Regrettably, the Nd:YAG 'dental laser' (free-running pulsed – 150 μs pulse width) was marketed as being suitable in tooth cavity preparation – a claim that was quickly deemed to be erroneous for clinical relevance. Early research into this claim supported the ablative effect of the 1,064 nm wavelength on accessible pigmented carious lesions,[1-3] but whenever healthy enamel and dentine was exposed to the laser energy, the comparatively long pulse width and associated heat transfer, combined with the lack of water spray, resulted in thermal cracking and melting of hydroxyapatite (Figs 1 and 2), together with high intra-pulpal temperatures, as investigated by a number of workers.[4-11] It is pertinent to note that thermal cracking is also evident with rotary instrumentation (Fig. 3).

Interestingly, it was discovered that the reformed, amorphous hydroxyapatite in post-laser sites was more resistant to acid dissolution and some studies were published advocating the use of the Nd:YAG laser in a quasi-fissure sealant technique for erupted posterior teeth.[12-16]

The carbon dioxide wavelength and emission mode (continuous or gated continuous wave) of commercially available lasers also made it impractical for restorative procedures (Figs 4-6). Although there is a high absorption peak of this wavelength (in the region of 10,000 nm) by carbonated hydroxyapatite (CHA), the continuous wave emission of laser energy and lack of axial water coolant resulted in carbonisation, cracking and melting of tooth tissue.[17-19] During laser light generation, the slow decay from the energised state in the CO_2 active medium results, potentially, in a number of individual wavelengths from this laser (9,300, 9,600, 10,300 and 10,600 nm). If one of the shorter wavelengths other than the usual 10,600 nm is selected, the absorption coefficient of CHA (carbonate group) increases greatly.[20,21] Featherstone

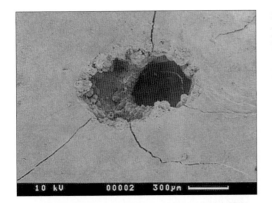

Fig. 1 Scanning electron micrograph (SEM) of enamel exposed to Nd:YAG laser energy, showing an ablation cavity surrounded by thermal cracking

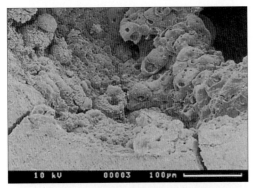

Fig. 2 Close up showing melted mineral structure of enamel

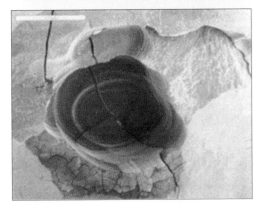

Fig. 3 SEM of rotary bur and enamel

and co-workers at UCSF (California, USA) have investigated extensively with an experimental ultra-pulsed 9,300 and 9,600 nm laser, the ablation rates of enamel and dentine, with much success. In addition, the removal, through ablation, of the carbonate group from the CHA molecule results in a greatly increased acid-resistant compound.[22-26]

The development of the Er:YAG and Er,Cr:YSGG lasers and investigations of their action on dental tissues shifted the emphasis from 'fringe' beneficial action of laser light towards a true ablation, that did not cause thermal or mechanical damage to the tooth or pulp and was sufficiently fast to be acceptable in a clinical setting.[27-29] The prime chromophore of the erbium YAG wavelength is water and the free-running micro-pulse emission mode results in rapid and expansive vaporisation (Fig. 7). When exposed to this wavelength, the small amounts of water contained in enamel and dentine are vaporised, causing an explosive dislocation of the gross structure (Figs 8-10).

Clinically, this is seen as ejection of micro-fragments of tooth tissue within the laser plume and the change in pressure in the immediately surrounding air results in an audible 'popping' sound. In target tissue that has greater water content (caries > dentine > enamel), the popping sound is louder. With experience, this can aid the clinician in selectively ablating carious vs non-carious tissue.[30] Compared to near-infrared wavelengths, the explosive outward effect of erbium laser energy results in minimal thermal diffusion through the tooth structure.

Co-axial with this laser is a water spray, to aid in dispersing ablation products and to provide cooling of the target site. This is vitally important as, in a situation of laser incident energy commensurate with tooth cutting, the ablation front will be in advance of the thermal front. Insufficient water coolant and consequent dispersal of ablation products during cavity preparation can lead to a build-up of eschar, which can become super-heated (Fig. 11). Conduction of this thermal energy to surrounding tooth tissue will lead to morphological cracking and melting, pain and possible pulpal damage.[31] An additional factor may be the shielding effect of the ejected debris and laser plume products into the line of the incident beam (Fig. 12).[32,33] The development of ultra-short pulse laser emissions of the erbium group of wavelengths appears promising in reducing the conductive heat potential, whilst increasing the rates of tissue ablation.

The other major laser wavelength that is applicable to tooth and bone ablation is the Er,Cr:YSGG (2,780 nm). This laser is similar to the Er:YAG in that it is absorbed by water and both wavelengths ablate through vaporisation of interstitial water,[34] although the absorption coefficient is slightly lower (4,000 cm^{-1} vs 13,000 cm^{-1} for Er:YAG). When one examines the absorption curve of CHA (enamel), there is a peak, coincident with 2,700 nm, representing absorption by the hydroxyl group (OH$^-$) contained in the mineral molecule (Fig. 13).

It is thought that the simultaneous ablation of this radical, with concomitant rapid heating of the mineral together with some direct vaporisation of whole water in hard tissue, contributes to the explosive dislocation of the target tissue when using this laser.[33] Claims have been made as to the involvement of the atomised water spray, used with the erbium YSGG and referred to as a hydrokinetic effect.[35] The hypothesis draws on the postulation that water droplets axial to the laser beam absorb kinetic energy and are accelerated to aid hard tissue ablation. Investigation into this effect has questioned the validity of such claims and in addition, with comparable incident energies, suggested that the ablation rate of the erbium YSGG with enamel is slightly slower than that of erbium YAG.[34] As mentioned above, this might be explained by the absorption dynamics of the YSGG and transfer of conductive heat from

LASERS IN DENTISTRY

Fig. 4 (left) Buccal cavity, lower canine

Fig. 5 (right) Following use of a carbon dioxide laser (10,600 nm). The erroneous use of this laser wavelength produced rapid carbonisation

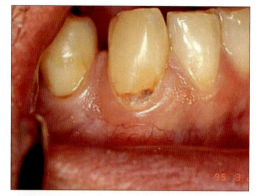
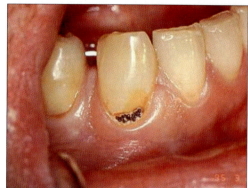

Fig. 6 (left) Restoration completed with hand instruments. Luckily, the tooth vitality was preserved, with no ill-effects

Fig. 7 (right) Er:YAG laser in use. Note non-contact mode of operation and disruption of water spray

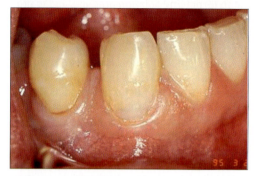
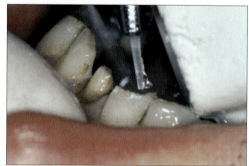

Fig. 8 (left) Buccal caries, LL 4

Fig. 9 (right) Following cavity preparation with Er:YAG 2,940 nm laser

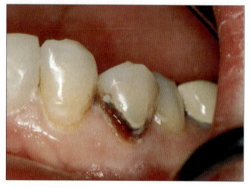
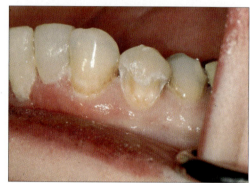

Fig. 10 (left) Completed restoration

Fig. 11 (right) Ablation cavities cut in tooth tissue. The small cavity on the right was cut with Er:YAG laser energy and co-axial water spray. The cavity to the left was cut with the Er:YAG laser without water and shows the carbonisation that readily develops

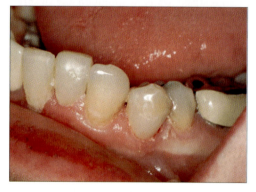
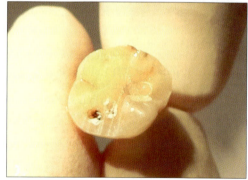

apatite to free water, although Walsh and Cummings have suggested that absorption of mid-infrared radiation by water is a function of temperature and pressure, both of which rise rapidly during an ablative laser pulse.[36] Apel *et al.* further confirmed this slight difference in their investigation into the ablation threshold of enamel with these lasers, finding values of 9-11 J cm^{-2} for Er:YAG and 10-14 J cm^{-2} for Er,Cr:YSGG.[37] Nonetheless, both laser wavelengths allow cavity preparation within acceptable clinical parameters.[38]

Early erbium lasers had rudimentary hand-pieces which were comparatively heavy. In addition, the delivery of laser energy through a non-contact sapphire window proved inaccurate in delivery of precise cutting action. Newer developments have resulted in balanced waveguides or low-OH$^-$ fibres, together with hand-pieces that are similar to turbines and use contact tips (Figs 14-17). Tissue ablation results from end-on emission of laser energy from the tip, which should be moved gently over the tooth surface to develop the cavity.

Numerous studies have been carried out to investigate the ablation rates of both wavelengths with enamel, dentine and caries,

SURGICAL LASERS

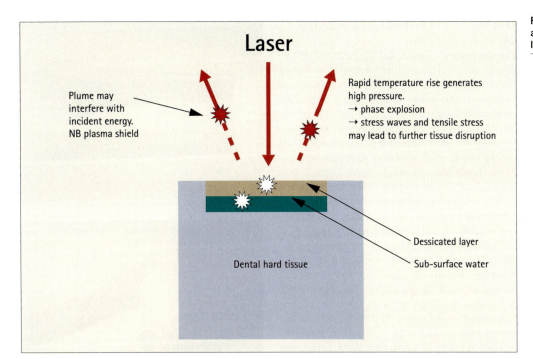

Fig. 12 Graphic showing the interactive zones between laser light, laser plume and tooth structure

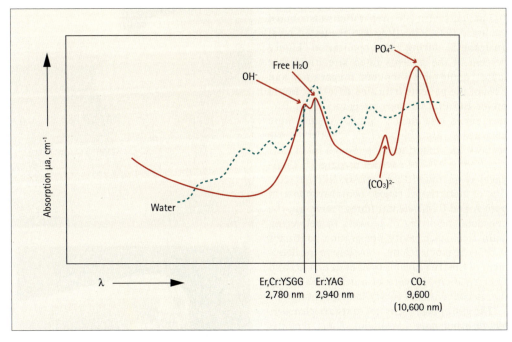

Fig. 13 Absorption curve of carbonated hydroxyapatite (CHA) interaction with Er,Cr:YSGG, Er:YAG and CO_2 laser wavelengths. Peaks at 2,700 nm and 2,900 nm correspond to OH^- group and free water; a small peak at approx 7,000 nm is coincident with $(CO_3)^{2-}$ group absorption; absorption at 9,600 nm is coincident with the phosphate group in the molecule; water absorption is shown as a dotted line. (Produced in conjunction with Prof. J. Featherstone, UCSF, California, USA)

together with non-metallic or non-thermofused ceramic restoratives such as direct composite resin and glass-ionomer cements (Figs 18-20). Under normal operating parameters, pulpal temperature has been shown to rise minimally (<5°C) during laser-assisted cavity preparation. Comparisons have been advantageously made between laser use and rotary instrumentation, although speed comparisons fall below that obtained with an airotor.

The gross and micro-appearance of a 'laser' cavity in tooth tissue is essentially a crater form (Fig. 21), which is markedly different to the 'classical' cavity form obtained with rotary instrumentation and consistent with the production of stable amalgam restorations.[39] However, the micro-dislocation of mineral at the cavity edges, visually evident as 'etched' in appearance, can be beneficially employed in aiding the bonding of composite resin materials (Fig. 22).

Studies carried out into the marginal integrity of such restorations reflect a poor stability, partly explained by a post-ablation weakness in marginal enamel.[40-42] Interestingly, one study comparing laser and bur preparation but both without acid etching, found that marginal integrity was greater following laser preparation.[43] However, when the cut surface is further treated with conventional acid-etch techniques, this improves the longevity of the restoration, with some enhanced bond-strength.[44,45] This facility can be employed as an adjunct where restorative procedures requiring facial or incisal bonding of direct composite resin materials is required, or in the placement of orthodontic brackets (Figs 23-26).

LASERS IN DENTISTRY

Fig. 14 Top: early Er:YAG hand-piece; bottom: current hand-piece, which is lighter and more accurate in use

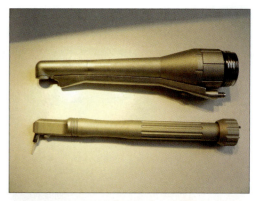

Fig. 15 Older (left) non-contact and newer (right) laser hand-piece with sapphire contact tip. The older head incorporates a flat sapphire window

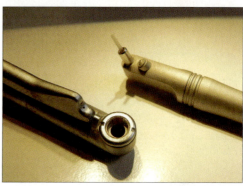

Fig. 16 'Old-style' hand-piece in use

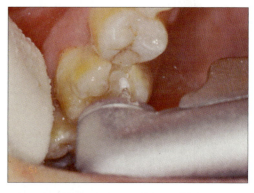

Fig. 17 Latest developments incorporate fibre-optics

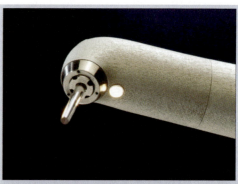

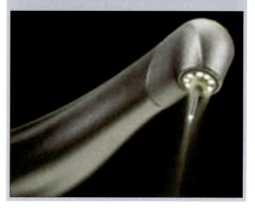

PAIN PERCEPTION DURING LASER-ASSISTED CAVITY PREPARATION

The avoidance of pain during restorative and dental surgical procedures remains a strong factor in promoting patient acceptance of treatment and many studies have been carried out to evaluate this.[46-51] The use of the Nd:YAG laser in developing pulpal analgesia, possibly through interference with the 'gate theory' of neural stimulus propagation, has been suggested, although investigation into the subjectivity or placebo effect has rendered its application inconsistent.[52-54]

Perhaps of greater significance in addressing claims of pain avoidance during laser-assisted tooth preparation is the lack of tactile and thermal stimulation compared to rotary instrumentation. In addition, there is the patient-centred factor of previous experience of turbine use together with other emotional and conditioning states. Many studies into the use of erbium lasers in restorative dentistry include reports of such treatment being less painful;[55-61] Keller and Hibst investigated 103 patients with 206 preparations distributed amongst 194 teeth. Only 6% requested local anaesthesia during laser application. Eighty percent of the patients rated laser treatment more comfortable than bur preparation and 82% of the patients indicated that they would prefer the Er:YAG laser preparation for further caries treatment.[62] Similar results were obtained by Matsumoto et al., reporting a 6% request for anaesthesia, although pain was reported in 32% of cavities prepared.[63] Chaiyavej et al. found that Er:YAG, like bur cutting of tooth tissue, caused neural response in both A and C intradental fibres.[64] Overall, the anecdotal reporting of prowess in delivering 'pain free' laser cavity preparation continues to provoke much debate – possibly to the detriment of the true capability of both Er:YAG and Er,Cr:YSGG in delivery of a genuine alternative to conventional rotary instrumentation.

'The aim of the wise is not to secure pleasure, but to avoid pain' (Aristotle). There remains the duty of the practitioner in showing professional responsibility towards the individual patient, their management and their comfort.

ERBIUM LASERS AND CAVITY PREPARATION
i) Enamel

Enamel is composed, by volume, of 85% mineral (predominately carbonated hydroxyapatite), 12% water and 3% organic proteins. The majority of free water exists within the peri-prismatic protein matrix. Of the major hard tissues, enamel exhibits greatest resistance to laser ablation and this is seen most in healthy, fluoridated, occlusal sites, where ablation rate is approximately 20% of that achieved with a turbine. Fluoridated enamel presents a greater resistance, due to the combined effects of a harder fluorapatite $(Ca_{10}(PO_4)_6F_2)$ mineral and the replacement of the hydroxyl group by fluoride (Fig. 27).

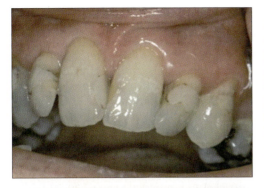
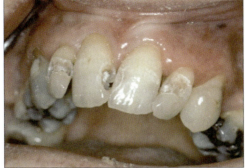
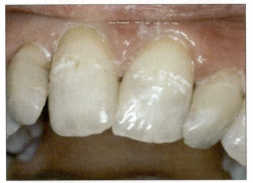
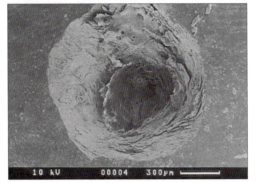
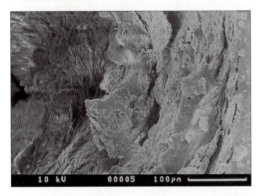

Fig. 18 (left) Multiple failing composite restorations

Fig. 19 (right) Er:YAG laser ablation of composite material

Fig. 20 (left) Completed new restorations

Fig. 21 (right) SEM of ablation cavity in enamel, Er:YAG laser

Fig. 22 High power SEM of laser-etched surface of enamel (Er:YAG 2,940 nm). Such margins should be further acid-etched to stabilise any weakened enamel fragments

In Class III, IV and V cavity sites and certainly where prismatic density is less (as in deciduous teeth), the ablation rate is comparable to rotary instrumentation.[65-67] Anecdotally, the speed of laser cutting is maximised if the incident beam is directed parallel to the prismatic structure and this is supportive of addressing the wavelength to the prime chromophore and its location within the tissue structure. In early research into the use of Er:YAG and enamel, it was shown that laser power parameters of approximately 350 mJ/2-4 pps (average power 0.7-1.4 W) would initiate enamel ablation in human teeth.[68] With the development of better co-axial coolant and shorter pulses, fast and efficient cavity preparation can be achieved with power levels of 400-700 mJ/10-20 pps (average power range 4-8 W) which, with adequate water cooling, does not cause pulpal damage. Clinical experience would suggest that with 'harder' occlusal enamel, the use of higher energy-per-pulse and lower repetition rates provides for easier ablation. Where an etch-bonding technique is required, lower power levels (350-500 mJ/5-10 pps - average power 1.75-3.5 W) should be employed. The concept of average power is more important in those lasers where the pulse rate is fixed.

ii) Dentine

Dentine has a higher water content and less mineral density than enamel, being 47% by volume mineral (carbonated hydroxyapatite), 33% protein (mostly collagen) and 20% water. Consequently, ablation rates are faster than for enamel and power parameters can be correspondingly lower (average power range 3-5 W) and it is essential to use co-axial water spray (Fig. 28).

The sound resonance is greater, reflecting the greater water content. With carious dentine there is a potential in gross caries for the laser beam to quickly pass through the surface layer, thus leading to dehydration in deeper layers. Where gross caries is present it is advisable to use an excavator to remove bulk volume, both to prevent heat damage and to expedite cavity preparation. Both erbium lasers will leave a cut surface without a smear layer and it is advisable to use a dentine protector on open tubules exposed by the ablation process (Figs 29-31).

ERBIUM LASERS AND BONE ABLATION

Early study into the effect of the Er:YAG laser on bone showed that, as with enamel and dentine ablation, tissue cutting is a thermally induced explosive process.[69,70] As with other hard tissue interaction, it is essential to maintain a co-axial water spray to prevent heat damage which would delay healing. Studies into the rate of thermal denaturation of collagen, a major component of bone tissue, show that above a critical temperature (74°C), the rate of collagen denaturation rapidly increases causing coagulation of tissue. Other forms of thermal damage and tissue necrosis follow similar kinetics.[71,72] At temperatures above 100-300°C there is an ascending dehydration, followed by carbonisation of proteins and lipids. The poor haemostatic effect of current mid-infrared lasers with adjunctive water spray, can be used to advantage in the ablation of bone, in ensuring blood perfusion of the surgical site (Figs 32 and 33).

However, the ablation process results in a considerable splatter of blood, and precautions (eye protection and mask) are recommended. An additional risk may be the creation of an air embolism in the tissue due to the air-induced water spray, although a review of the literature has not revealed any association. The acoustic level of bone ablation (100-120 dB) is much higher than with tooth tissue ablation.[73]

The use of erbium lasers in dento-alveolar surgery represents a less traumatic experience for the patient, when compared to the intense vibration of the slow-speed surgical bur. Ablation threshold measurements of 10-30 J cm^{-2} have been recorded for bone of varying density[74] and clinically, with maxillary alveolar bone, the speed of laser cutting is comparable with that of a bur and is slightly slower in the mandible, reflecting the greater cortical bone composition. It is considered important that excessive power parameters are avoided, to reduce the 'stall-out' effect of debris and minimise blood spatter. Laser power values of 350-500 mJ/10-20 pps (average power range 3.5-7.0 W) with maximal water spray appear to effect good ablation rates.

The micro-analysis of the cut surface (Figs 34-36) reveals little evidence of thermal damage and any char layer appears to be restricted to a minimal zone of 20-30 μm in depth.[74,75] Studies into the healing of lased bone would support the contention that the reduced physical trauma, reduced heating effects and reduced bacterial contamination, together with some claims to an osteogenic potential, lead to uncomplicated healing processes when compared to conventional use of a surgical bur.[76-80]

CONCLUSION

It is unquestioned that the patient avoidance of restorative dentistry is based upon the perceived association of such procedures with pain. Local anaesthetic drugs and

Fig. 23 (left) A decision was made to restore this tooth with a direct, acid-etch composite resin veneer

Fig. 24 (righth) Er:YAG 2,940 nm laser used to remove existing composite filling and to laser etch the labial surface

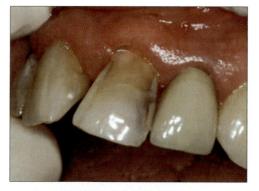
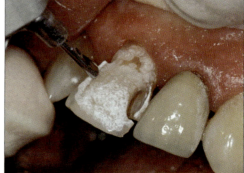

Fig. 25 (left) Finished restoration

Fig. 26 (right) For interstitial access, a dulled metal matrix can be used to prevent laser damage to the adjacent tooth surface

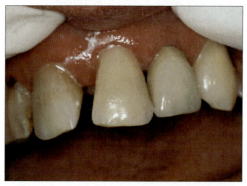
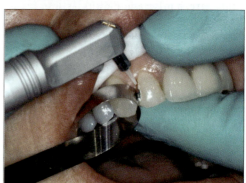

Fig. 27 Er:YAG laser ablation of occlusal enamel and cross-section to show depth of penetration

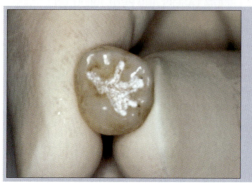
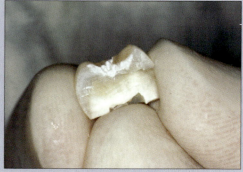

SURGICAL LASERS

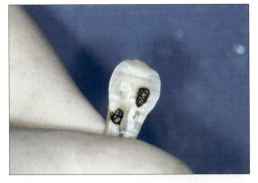
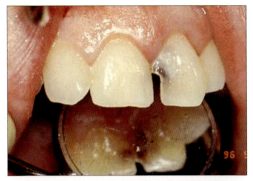

Fig. 28 (left) Vertical section of tooth showing laser use on dentine. Upper left area achieved with Er:YAG laser and water, upper right and lower left areas show Er:YAG and CO_2 laser wavelengths without water

Fig. 29 (right) Mesial carious cavity, UL 1

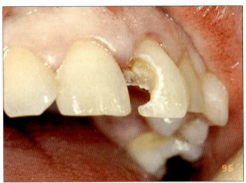
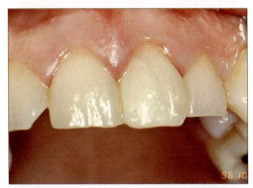

Fig. 30 (left) Er:YAG 2,940 nm laser used to define cavity, ablate caries and create a 'laser etch' on enamel margins

Fig. 31 (right) Finished restoration

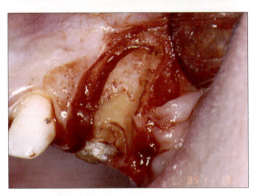
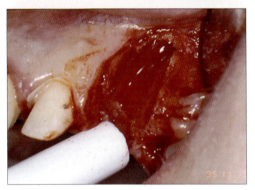

Fig. 32 (left) An Er:YAG 2,940 nm laser has been used to cut through the buccal plate of bone

Fig. 33 (right) Following removal of the root, note the accuracy of the cut and the free flow of blood

techniques can address the demands on delivery of care, but the emergence of many innovative mechanical and chemical modalities for tooth cavity preparation and caries control during the last 15 years bears testimony to a desire to find a clinically acceptable replacement to the dental turbine. This is not just a cosmetic exercise, as the risks of pulpal temperature rise and iatrogenic healthy tooth tissue damage, together with the sensory effects of sound and vibration associated with the dental turbine, have been investigated and acknowledged for many years. With this in mind, it is of little comfort that the rates of tissue ablation with rotary instrumentation remain faster than the alternatives. The wide application of current commercially-available laser wavelengths that have been shown to be safe within correct power parameters, endorses their incorporation into the armamentarium of the restorative and surgical dentist. With the rapidly-growing concept of early intervention of caries, together with the general move away from direct metal restorative material and an embracing of 'non-classical' micro-retentive tooth cavities, there is a strong argument that laser-assisted cavity preparation, caries control and bonding techniques will find growing acceptance.

The assistance provided by Professor J. Featherstone, UCSF, California, USA in the design of Figure 13 (absorption curve of CHA) is acknowledged.

1. Birardi V, Bossi L, Dinoi C. Use of the Nd:YAG laser in the treatment of early childhood caries. *Eur J Paediatr Dent* 2004; **5:** 98-101.
2. Bassi G, Chawla S, Patel M. The Nd:YAG laser in caries removal. *Br Dent J* 1994; **177:** 248-250.
3. Harris D M, White J M, Goodis H *et al.* Selective ablation of surface enamel caries with a pulsed Nd:YAG dental laser. *Lasers Surg Med* 2002; **30:** 342-350.
4. Cox C J, Pearson G J, Palmer G. Preliminary in vitro investigation of the effects of pulsed Nd:YAG laser radiation on enamel and dentine. *Biomaterials* 1994; **15:** 1145-1151.
5. Yamada M K, Uo M, Ohkawa S, Akasaka T, Watari F. Three-dimensional topographic scanning electron microscope and Raman spectroscopic analyses of the irradiation effect on teeth by Nd:YAG, Er:YAG, and CO_2 lasers. *J Biomed Mater Res B Appl Biomater* 2004; **71:** 7-15.
6. Yamada M K, Watari F. Imaging and non-contact profile analysis of Nd:YAG laser-irradiated teeth by scanning electron microscopy and confocal laser scanning microscopy. *Dent Mater J* 2003; **22:** 556-568.
7. Srimaneepong V, Palamara J E, Wilson P R. Pulpal space pressure and temperature changes from Nd:YAG laser irradiation of dentin. *J Dent* 2002; **30:** 291-296.
8. Lan W H, Chen K W, Jeng J H, Lin C P, Lin S K. A comparison of the morphological changes after Nd-YAG and CO_2 laser irradiation of dentin surfaces. *J Endod* 2000; **26:** 450-453.

LASERS IN DENTISTRY

Fig. 34 (left) SEM of bone cut with Er:YAG 2,940 nm laser

Fig. 35 (right) SEM of bone cut with surgical bur. Note smearing and thermal cracking

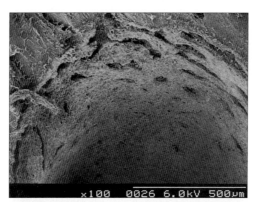
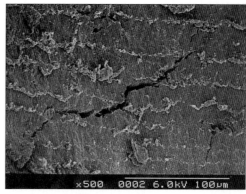

Fig. 36 SEM of bone exposed to Nd:YAG 1,064 nm laser, showing voids and re-formed melted mineral

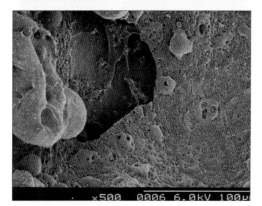

9. McDonald A, Claffey N, Pearson G, Blau W, Setchell D. The effect of Nd:YAG pulse duration on dentine crater depth. *J Dent* 2001; **29:** 43-53.
10. Goodis H E, White J M, Marshall G W Jr et al. Effects of Nd: and Ho:yttrium-aluminium-garnet lasers on human dentine fluid flow and dental pulp-chamber temperature in vitro. *Arch Oral Biol* 1997; **42:** 845-854.
11. Seka W, Fried D, Featherstone J D, Borzillary S F. Light deposition in dental hard tissue and simulated thermal response. *J Dent Res* 1995; **74:** 1086-1092.
12. Kwon Y H, Kwon O W, Kim H I, Kim K H. Nd:YAG laser ablation and acid resistance of enamel. *Dent Mater J* 2003; **22:** 404-411.
13. Tsai C L, Lin Y T, Huang S T, Chang H W. In vitro acid resistance of CO_2 and Nd-YAG laser-treated human tooth enamel. *Caries Res* 2002; **36:** 423-429.
14. Harazaki M, Hayakawa K, Fukui T, Isshiki Y, Powell L G. The Nd-YAG laser is useful in prevention of dental caries during orthodontic treatment. *Bull Tokyo Dent Coll* 2001; **42:** 79-86.
15. Hossain M, Nakamura Y, Kimura Y, Yamada Y, Kawanaka T, Matsumoto K. Effect of pulsed Nd:YAG laser irradiation on acid demineralization of enamel and dentin. *J Clin Laser Med Surg* 2001; **19:** 105-108.
16. Myaki S I, Watanabe I S, Eduardo C de P, Issao M. Nd:YAG laser effects on the occlusal surface of premolars. *Am J Dent* 1998; **11:** 103-105.
17. Malmstrom H S, McCormack S M, Fried D, Featherstone J D. Effect of CO_2 laser on pulpal temperature and surface morphology: an in vitro study. *J Dent* 2001; **29:** 521-529.
18. Watanabe I, Lopes R A, Brugnera A, Katayama A Y, Gardini A E. Effect of CO_2 laser on class V cavities of human molar teeth under a scanning electron microscope. *Braz Dent J* 1996; **7:** 27-31.
19. Friedman S, Liu M, Izawa T, Moynihan M, Dorscher-Kim J, Kim S. Effects of CO_2 laser irradiation on pulpal blood flow. *Proc Finn Dent Soc* 1992; **88 (Suppl 1):** 167-171.
20. Konishi N, Fried D, Staninec M, Featherstone J D. Artificial caries removal and inhibition of artificial secondary caries by pulsed CO_2 laser irradiation. *Am J Dent* 1999; **12:** 213-216.
21. Mullejans R, Eyrich G, Raab W H, Frentzen M. Cavity preparation using a superpulsed 9.6-microm CO_2 laser – a histological investigation. *Lasers Surg Med* 2002; **30:** 331-336.
22. Featherstone J D, Barrett-Vespone N A, Fried D, Kantorowitz Z, Seka W. CO_2 laser inhibitor of artificial caries-like lesion progression in dental enamel. *J Dent Res* 1998; **77:** 1397-1403.
23. Kantorowitz Z, Featherstone J D, Fried D. Caries prevention by CO_2 laser treatment: dependency on the number of pulses used. *J Am Dent Assoc* 1998; **129:** 585-591.
24. Goodis H E, Fried D, Gansky S, Rechmann P, Featherstone J D. Pulpal safety of 9.6 microm TEA CO_2 laser used for caries prevention. *Lasers Surg Med* 2004; **35:** 104-110.
25. McCormack S M, Fried D, Featherstone J D, Glena R E, Seka W. Scanning electron microscope observations of CO_2 laser effects on dental enamel. *J Dent Res* 1995; **74:** 1702-1708.
26. Tepper S A, Zehnder M, Pajarola G F, Schmidlin P R. Increased fluoride uptake and acid resistance by CO_2 laser-irradiation through topically applied fluoride on human enamel in vitro. *J Dent* 2004; **32:** 635-641.
27. Takamori K, Furukawa H, Morikawa Y, Katayama T, Watanabe S. Basic study on vibrations during tooth preparations caused by high-speed drilling and Er:YAG laser irradiation. *Lasers Surg Med* 2003; **32:** 25-31.
28. Glockner K, Rumpler J, Ebeleseder K, Stadtler P. Intrapulpal temperature during preparation with the Er:YAG laser compared to the conventional burr: an in vitro study. *J Clin Laser Med Surg* 1998; **16:** 153-157.
29. Pelagalli J, Gimbel C B, Hansen R T, Swett A, Winn DW 2nd. Investigational study of the use of Er:YAG laser versus dental drill for caries removal and cavity preparation – phase I. *J Clin Laser Med Surg* 1997; **15:** 109-115.
30. Clark J, Symons A L, Diklic S, Walsh L J. Effectiveness of diagnosing residual caries with various methods during cavity preparation using conventional methods, chemo-mechanical caries removal, and Er:YAG laser. *Aust Dent J* 2001; **46 (Suppl):** S20.
31. Lee B S, Lin C P, Hung Y L, Lan W H. Structural changes of Er:YAG laser irradiated human dentin. *Photomed Laser Surg* 2004; **22:** 330-334.
32. Murray A K, Dickinson M R. High-speed photography of plasma during excimer laser-tissue interaction. *Phys Med Biol* 2004; **49:** 3325-3340.
33. Fried D. IR laser ablation of dental enamel. *Proc SPIE* 2000; **3910:** 136-148.
34. Freiberg R J, Cozean C D. Pulsed erbium laser ablation of hard dental tissue: the effects of atomized water spray versus water surface film. *Proc SPIE* 2002; **4610:** 74-84.
35. Riziou I, Kimmel A. *Atomized fluid particles for electro-magnetically induced cutting*. US Patent 5,741,247. 1998.
36. Walsh J T Jr, Cummings J P. Effect of the dynamic optical properties of water on midinfrared laser ablation. *Lasers Surg Med* 1994; **15:** 295-305.
37. Apel C, Meister J, Ioana R S, Franzen R, Hering P, Gutknecht N. The ablation threshold of Er:YAG and Er:YSGG laser radiation in dental enamel. *Lasers Med Sci* 2002; **17:** 246-252.
38. Harashima T, Kinoshita J, Kimura Y et al. Morphological comparative study on ablation of dental hard tissues at cavity preparation by Er:YAG and Er,Cr:YSGG lasers. *Photomed Laser Surg* 2005; **23:** 52-55.
39. Boyde A. Enamel structure and cavity margins. *Oper Dent* 1976; **1:** 13-28.
40. Chinelatti M A, Ramos R P, Chimello D T, Borsatto M C, Pecora J D, Palma-Dibb R G. Influence of the use of Er:YAG laser for cavity preparation and surface treatment in microleakage of resin-modified glass ionomer restorations. *Oper Dent* 2004; **29:** 430-436.
41. Corona S A, Borsatto M C, Pecora JD, De SA Rocha R A, Ramos T S, Palma-Dibb R G. Assessing microleakage of different class V restorations after Er:YAG laser and bur preparation. *J Oral Rehabil* 2003; **30:** 1008-1014.
42. Corona S A, Borsatto M, Dibb R G, Ramos R P, Brugnera A,

Pecora J D. Microleakage of class V resin composite restorations after bur, air-abrasion or Er:YAG laser preparation. *Oper Dent* 2001; **26:** 491-497.
43. Kohara E K, Hossain M, Kimura Y, Matsumoto K, Inoue M, Sasa R. Morphological and microleakage studies of the cavities prepared by Er:YAG laser irradiation in primary teeth. *J Clin Laser Med Surg* 2002; **20:** 141-147.
44. Niu W, Eto J N, Kimura Y, Takeda F H, Matsumoto K. A study on microleakage after resin filling of class V cavities prepared by Er:YAG laser. *J Clin Laser Med Surg* 1998; **16:** 227-231.
45. Gutknecht N, Apel C, Schafer C, Lampert F. Microleakage of composite fillings in Er,Cr:YSGG laser-prepared class II cavities. *Lasers Surg Med* 2001; **28:** 371-374.
46. Malamed S F. Pain and anxiety control in dentistry. *J Calif Dent Assoc* 1993; **21:** 35-38, 40-41.
47. Penfold C N. Pain-free oral surgery. *Dent Update* 1993; **20:** 421-426.
48. Maskell R. Pain-free dental treatment is changing dentistry's image. *Probe (Lond)* 1991; **33(9):** 36-37.
49. Arora R. Influence of pain-free dentistry and convenience of dental office on the choice of a dental practitioner: an experimental investigation. *Health Mark Q* 1999; **16(3):** 43-54.
50. Blechman A M. Pain-free and mobility-free orthodontics? *Am J Orthod Dentofacial Orthop* 1998; **113:** 379-383.
51. Delfino J. Public attitudes toward oral surgery: results of a Gallup poll. *J Oral Maxillofac Surg* 1997; **55:** 564-567.
52. Whitters C J, Hall A, Creanor S L et al. A clinical study of pulsed Nd:YAG laser-induced pulpal analgesia. *J Dent* 1995; **23:** 145-150.
53. Orchardson R, Whitters C J. Effect of HeNe and pulsed Nd:YAG laser irradiation on intradental nerve responses to mechanical stimulation of dentine. *Lasers Surg Med* 2000; **26:** 241-249.
54. Orchardson R, Peacock J M, Whitters C J. Effect of pulsed Nd:YAG laser radiation on action potential conduction in isolated mammalian spinal nerves. *Lasers Surg Med* 1997; **21:** 142-148.
55. Hubbard L G. Smile improvement: the laser way. *Dent Today* 2000; **19(2):** 94-95.
56. Smith T A, Thompson J A, Lee W E. Assessing patient pain during dental laser treatment. *J Am Dent Assoc* 1993; **124:** 90-95.
57. Kato J, Moriya K, Jayawardena J A, Wijeyeweera R L. Clinical application of Er:YAG laser for cavity preparation in children. *J Clin Laser Med Surg* 2003; **21:** 151-155.
58. Hadley J, Young D A, Eversole L R, Gornbein J A. A laser-powered hydrokinetic system for caries removal and cavity preparation. *J Am Dent Assoc* 2000; **131:** 777-785.
59. Dostalova T, Jelinkova H, Kucerova H et al. Noncontact Er:YAG laser ablation: clinical evaluation. *J Clin Laser Med Surg* 1998; **16:** 273-282.
60. Matsumoto K, Nakamura Y, Mazeki K, Kimura Y. Clinical dental application of Er:YAG laser for class V cavity preparation. *J Clin Laser Med Surg* 1996; **14:** 123-127.
61. Keller U, Hibst R. Effects of Er:YAG laser in caries treatment: a clinical pilot study. *Lasers Surg Med* 1997; **20:** 32-38.
62. Keller U, Hibst R, Geurtsen W et al. Erbium:YAG laser application in caries therapy. Evaluation of patient perception and acceptance. *J Dent* 1998; **26:** 649-656.
63. Matsumoto K, Hossain M, Hossain M M, Kawano H, Kimura Y. Clinical assessment of Er,Cr:YSGG laser application for cavity preparation. *J Clin Laser Med Surg* 2002; **20:** 17-21.
64. Chaiyavej S, Yamamoto H, Takeda A, Suda H. Response of feline intradental nerve fibers to tooth cutting by Er:YAG laser. *Lasers Surg Med* 2000; **27:** 341-349.
65. Stock K, Hibst R, Keller U. Comparison of Er:YAG and Er:YSGG laser ablation of dental hard tissues. *Proc SPIE* 2000; **3192:** 88-95.
66. Belikov A V, Erofeev A V, Shumilin V V, Tkachuk A M. Comparative study of the 3um laser action on different hard tissue samples using free running pulsed Er-doped YAG, YSGG, YAP and YLF lasers. *Proc SPIE* 1993; **2080:** 60-67.
67. Mercer C, Anderson P, Davis G. Sequential 3D X-ray microtomographic measurement of enamel and dentine ablation by an Er:YAG laser. *Br Dent J* 2003; **194:** 99-104.
68. Hibst R, Keller U. Mechanism of Er:YAG laser-induced ablation of dental hard substances. *Proc SPIE* 1993; **1880:** 156-162.
69. Hibst R. Mechanical effects of erbium:YAG laser bone ablation. *Lasers Surg Med* 1992; **12:** 125-130.
70. Peavy G M, Reinisch L, Payne J T, Venugopalan V. Comparison of cortical bone ablations by using infrared laser wavelengths 2.9 to 9.2 microm. *Lasers Surg Med* 1999; **25:** 421-434.
71. Thomsen S. Pathologic analysis of photothermal and photomechanical effects of laser-tissue interactions. *Photochem Photobiol* 1991; **53:** 825-835.
72. Thomsen S, Cheong W, Pearce J. Changes in collagen birefringence: a quantitative histologic marker of thermal damage in skin. *Proc SPIE* 1992; **1422:** 32-42.
73. Li Z Z, Reinisch L, Van de Merwe W P. Bone ablation with Er:YAG and CO_2 laser: study of thermal and acoustic effects. *Lasers Surg Med* 1992; **12:** 79-85.
74. Fried N M, Fried D. Comparison of Er:YAG and 9.6-microm TE CO_2 lasers for ablation of skull tissue. *Lasers Surg Med* 2001; **28:** 335-343.
75. Sasaki K M, Aoki A, Ichinose S, Ishikawa I. Ultrastructural analysis of bone tissue irradiated by Er:YAG laser. *Lasers Surg Med* 2002; **31:** 322-332.
76. Wang X, Zhang C, Matsumoto K. In vivo study of the healing processes that occur in the jaws of rabbits following perforation by an Er,Cr:YSGG laser. *Lasers Med Sci* 2005; **20:** 21-27.
77. Walsh J T Jr, Deutsch T F. Er:YAG laser ablation of tissue: measurement of ablation rates. *Lasers Surg Med* 1989; **9:** 327-337.
78. Wang X, Ishizaki N T, Suzuki N, Kimura Y, Matsumoto K. Morphological changes of bovine mandibular bone irradiated by Er,Cr:YSGG laser: an in vitro study. *J Clin Laser Med Surg* 2002; **20:** 245-250.
79. Pourzarandian A, Watanabe H, Aoki A et al. Histological and TEM examination of early stages of bone healing after Er:YAG laser irradiation. *Photomed Laser Surg* 2004; **22:** 342-350.
80. O'Donnell R J, Deutsch T F, Flotte R J et al. Effect of Er:YAG laser holes on osteoinduction in demineralized rat calvarial allografts. *J Orthop Res* 1996; **14:** 108-113.

IN BRIEF

- Regulation of laser use is similar to that employed for X-radiation.
- The prime risk is associated with the unprotected eye. Damage can be instantaneous and permanent. All lasers are classified according to this risk.
- Regulation in the UK is through the Healthcare Commission in the implementation of internationally-accepted guidelines as to all aspects of laser safety in the dental surgery.
- It is the responsibility of all clinicians undertaking laser dentistry to observe safe practice and, where required, register such use with regulatory authorities.

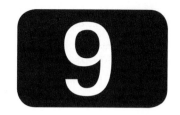

Laser regulation and safety in general dental practice

Laser devices, instruments and machines vary in their potential for light energy emission from low-powered hand-held or integrated devices, to high-powered units capable of cutting and ablating tissue and materials. The safe use of lasers in dentistry extends to all personnel who might be exposed, either deliberately or by accident, and demands of the lead clinician an approach to their use in order that risk of accidental exposure to laser light is minimised. The scope for regulations extends in similar ways to those imposed on the use of ionising radiation in the dental practice. Laser safety measures in the dental surgery are often drawn from the safe approach to the use of lasers in general and other specialties in medicine and surgery. This chapter serves to examine the risks involved in laser use in dentistry, the regulations governing safe use and the responsibilities of personnel involved in providing treatment to patients.

LASERS IN DENTISTRY

1. Introduction, history of lasers and laser light production
2. Laser-tissue interaction
3. Low-level laser use in dentistry
4. Lasers and soft tissue: 'loose' soft tissue surgery
5. Lasers and soft tissue: 'fixed' soft tissue surgery
6. Lasers and soft tissue: periodontal therapy
7. Surgical laser use in implantology and endodontics
8. Surgical lasers and hard dental tissue
9. **Laser regulation and safety in general dental practice**

REGULATIONS AS TO USE OF LASERS IN DENTISTRY

As described earlier, the expansive development of laser use in medicine and surgery occurred during the 1970s and early 1980s. In the UK, sufficient concern was raised as to the suitability of training and regulation of practitioners using lasers, which resulted in a timely amendment to the Nursing Homes Act in 1985. Although laser use was considered peripheral to the core of the Act, compulsory registration of medical (and, after 1990, dental) practitioners with local health authorities was required, in addition to a general compliance under the Health and Safety Act. With respect to dental practice, the new 'laser dentists' using surgical lasers received perfunctory inspection from health authority personnel. Although the auspices of the Nursing Homes Act were expansive, dental practice inspection was often limited to an assessment by a laser protection advisor (usually a medical physicist), as to the suitability of premises, controlled area, local rules and training record of dentists using these lasers.

In 2000, the Nursing Homes Act was replaced by the Care Standards Act and the setting up of the Healthcare Commission in 2004[1] has resulted in a much more specific attitude to the regulation of all personnel who use both lasers and intense light sources. Notwithstanding the extent of the scope of interest shown by this authority towards the provision of primary healthcare in general, and the implications for general dental practitioners who use lasers, specifically the duty of the practitioner, in using surgical lasers can be listed as follows:

- Application for registration as a user of a surgical laser with the Healthcare Commission
- Demonstration of physical barriers to safeguard safety – controlled area, limited access
- Demonstration of training received by all involved in laser use, local rules, and a record of laser use
- Demonstration of suitability of laser for clinical use, machine maintenance, and laser safety eye protection
- Recording and audit of unwanted effects associated with laser use.

In contrast to other countries, there is as yet no statutory requirement *per se* for formal

	Short time exposure (t)		Long time exposure (T)		Specular reflection of beam	Skin exposure to beam
	Magnified exposure	Unprotected eye	Magnified exposure	Unprotected eye		
I	✓	✓	✓	✓	✓	✓
IM	✹	✓	✹	✓	✓	✓
II	✓	✓	✹	✹	✓	✓
IIM	✹	✓	✹	✹	✓	✓
IIIR	⚠	⚠	✹	✹	✓	✓
IIIB	✹	✹	✹	✹	⚠	⚠
IV	✹	✹	✹	✹	✹	✹

✓ No risk from exposure to laser beam

⚠ Caution required to prevent exposure to beam

✹ Maximal protection required. Laser beam is dangerous

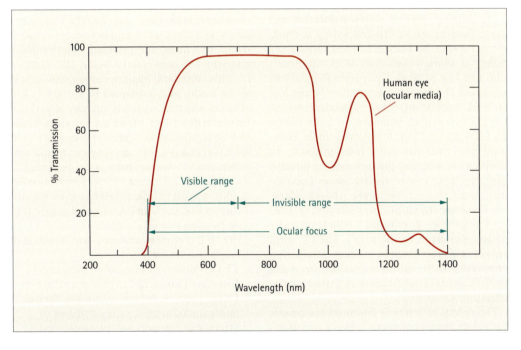

Fig. 1 Risk analysis relative to tissue and laser class

Fig. 2 Illustration of the transmissive (inverse of absorption) nature of visible and near-infrared wavelengths through the cornea, lens and associated structures. Above 1,400 nm, there is increased absorption by the water content of these structures

or on-going training or education in the use of lasers in dentistry in the UK. The Healthcare Commission would view attendance at postgraduate courses, such as those offered by the European Society for Oral Laser Applications (ESOLA) and the Academy of Laser Dentistry (ALD), as being indicative of on-going training and proficiency examinations given by such organisations are accepted by the Healthcare Commission as evidence of the suitability of the practitioner to use surgical lasers on patients.

The specifics of safety with regard to the use of lasers extend primarily to eye protection, although target oral tissue exposure is important; the parallel requirements of regulations with regard to ionising radiation equipment can be readily appreciated.

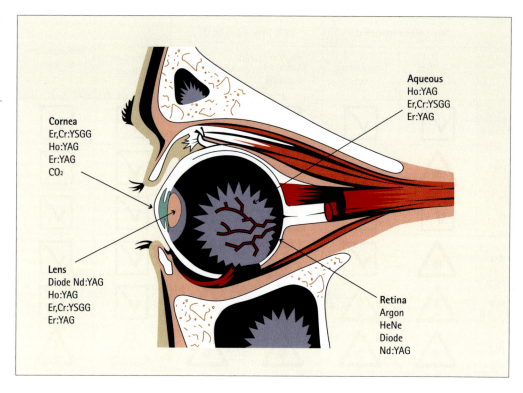

Fig. 3 Wavelength/site risk analysis of the eye. Non-pigmented structures towards the front of the eye will be most at risk from longer wavelengths, whereas retinal structures are at risk from short infrared and visible wavelengths

LEGAL ASPECTS OF LASER USE IN DENTAL PRACTICE

The first guidelines were issued in the 1960s, by defence research organisations in the US and the UK, and then by the American Conference of Governmental Industrial Hygienists.[2] However, with regard to any laser used in dental practice, as in any healthcare establishment, general safety legislation will apply, such as the Health and Safety at Work, etc Act 1974, the Management of Health and Safety at Work Regulations 1999, the Provision and Use of Work Equipment Regulations 1998 and the Personal Protective Equipment at Work Regulations 1992.[3] Compliance with the current British Standard on laser safety, BS EN 60825-1:1994, is required under European directives for many laser products. In addition, as with any product sold for medical use, any laser sold in the European Community must carry a 'CE' mark (the CE Marking Directive 93/68/EEC was adopted in 1993 – 'Conformité Européene', which literally means 'European conformity'). The CE mark proves to buyers that the product (production prototype) fulfils all the essential safety and environmental requirements as defined in the European directives.

The safety of lasers is based on the proper design of laser equipment and on the adoption of appropriate precautions during use. What discrepancy that might have occurred between the policies adopted by the USA and North America and other major regions, has been somewhat unified through the definition and adoption of the recommendations of the International Electro-technical Commission (IEC). This has resulted in a broad set of regulations that safeguard the product licence of laser machines and define protection measures for personnel who are associated with their use. Detailed requirements are given in a number of recognised safety standards, the principal international standard for laser safety being IEC 60825-1.[4] This standard applies throughout much of the world, and is adopted in Europe as EN 60825-1, where it is used in support of various European directives.[5] The USA has always had its own regulation on lasers (known as 21 CFR 1040.10); this is a USA government regulation (rather than a standard) and is written into US law. However, the issue of FDA Laser Notice 50 in 2001, sought to inform laser product manufacturers that the US FDA will now accept IEC classification and labelling.

The IEC recommendations are expanded through two instruments:

1. CE ('Conformité Européene') Marking Directive (93/68/EEC) 1993 Laser Product Licence, which defines suitability for use, clinical parameters, safety features of lasers, environment safety, patient safety, LSO, laser protection advisor, administrative code, record keeping and laser maintenance
2. IEC (EN) 60825-1:2001 *Safety of laser products part 1: equipment classification, requirements and user's guide*, which defines laser classes and measurement conditions, labelling, engineering controls etc, maximum permissible exposures (MPE) and accessible emission limits (AEL).

Table 1 Laser classification pre- and post- IEC (EN) 60825-1. Alignment of columns indicates relationship between the old classes and new

Pre-2002	I		II		IIIA	IIIB	IV
Post-2002	I	1M	II	2M	IIIR	IIIB	IV

REGULATION

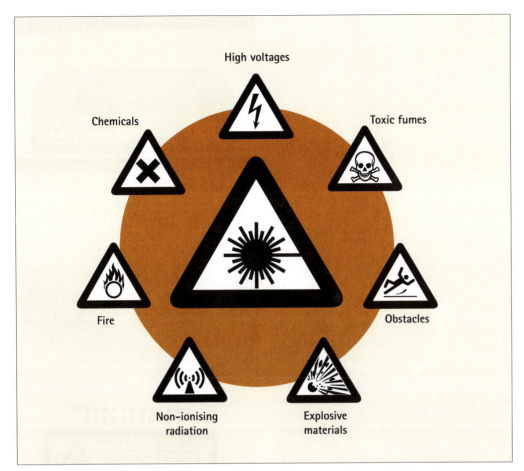

Fig. 4 The potential risks posed by surgical lasers within the clinical workplace. Source: Health Protection Agency UK

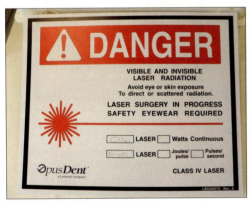

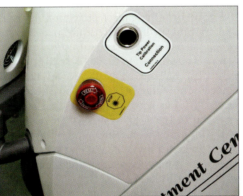

Fig. 5 (left) Laser warning sign, wavelength designated

Fig. 6 (right) Emergency 'STOP' button

Within the UK, the regulation of practices wishing to use surgical and other powerful lasers is undertaken by the Healthcare Commission, which draws upon legislation outlined above in its determination of safe and proper use. The Healthcare Commission has taken over the work of The National Care Standards Commission in ensuring compliance with the Care Standards Act 2000, which denotes national minimum standards for laser use. Dental practices using powerful lasers (Class 4 – see below) must register with the Healthcare Commission.[6]

LASER CLASSIFICATION

Originally, the classification of lasers used in healthcare was through an ascending Class I-Class IV to denote increased risk associated with use, and this classification is still in operation in the USA (I, IIA, II, IIIA, IIIB and IV). In the light of IEC recommendations, such classification has been revised to reflect exposure during use with magnification instruments, such as surgical microscopes. An overview of the classes of lasers, which represents their essential power, is given in Table 1.

The classification recognises risks associated with laser use and hazards pertaining to exposure of the eye and other tissues to the laser beam.[7-9] A 'worst case' scenario is adopted, which includes minimal distance from the laser, prolonged exposure to laser light and an assumption that non-protective spectacles are worn. Lasers have to be properly labelled to indicate their class and to warn users of their potential hazard. They must also incorporate certain safety features, dependent on their class, which are specified in the safety standard.

LASERS IN DENTISTRY

Fig. 7 Ports for foot-pedal and fibre

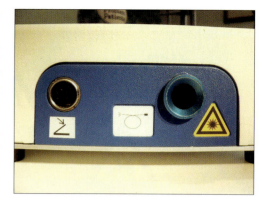

Fig. 8 Backplate, diode 810 nm laser, showing service port, remote interlock port and mains electricity socket (fused)

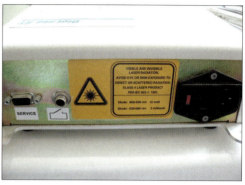

Fig. 9 Back-plate, Er:YAG/CO_2 laser

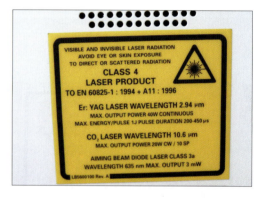

Fig. 10 Backplate, Er:YAG/CO_2 laser showing mains supply ports

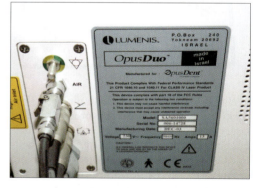

Fig. 11 Designated delivery system with unique interlock/wavelength

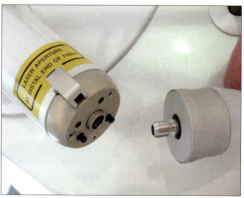

In 2002, a revision in accordance with European Standard EN 60825-1 was undertaken, with respect to maximum permissible exposure levels (MPEs), which rendered the adoption of the new classification. Individual MPE values vary according to the varying sensitivity of possible target tissues, eg the eye and skin and are expressed in Joules or Watts per area (J cm^{-2}, W cm^{-2}).[10] Generally, the longer the wavelength, the higher the MPE value; the longer the exposure time, the lower the MPE value.

Classes of laser

Class I: examples are found in CD players and laser caries detectors. Viewing with the naked eye poses no implicit risk, but caution should be observed if wearing spectacles or using optical devices (Class IM – 'magnifying'). The maximum power output of these lasers is 40 µW (blue light) and 400 µW for red light emissions.

Class II: examples are laser pointers. There exist specific risks to viewing light emissions, both to the naked eye and when using magnification.[11,12] The maximum output is 1 mW.

Class III: the 'old' Class IIIA is replaced by Classes IM and IIM. Class IIIB represents maximal power output of 0.5 W. Examples include 'soft' medical lasers (LLLT), laser light show equipment and laser measuring devices. Environmental controls, protective eyewear, appointment of assigned safety personnel (laser safety officer, laser protection advisor) and training in laser safety are required by personnel using these lasers.[13]

A new classification is the Class IIIR, which may also include some low level medical devices and targeting lasers, but generally lasers of lower power outputs than IIIA. For emission in the visual range of wavelengths (400-700 nm), the maximum power output is 5 mW and with invisible wavelengths, 2 mW. The same safety measures are required as with Class IIIB lasers.[14]

Class IV: This Class includes all high-powered, surgical and other cutting lasers. There is no upper limit of power output. All surgical lasers used in dentistry and oral and maxillofacial surgery are included. The protective measures applicable to Class III lasers are further endorsed with the additional risk of fire hazards, due to flash-point temperatures being reached in chemicals used adjunctively to surgical procedures. This group of lasers represents the greatest risk of damage, both to unprotected persons and target tissue, either through direct or reflected and scattered beams.[15]

The new grouping classification can be used to define the broader risks associated with inadvertent use. The greater aspects of laser safety for unprotected personnel can be grouped as instantaneous eye exposure, longer (magnified) eye exposure, direct or specular reflected beam exposure and skin (non-occular) exposure. The relative risks

REGULATION

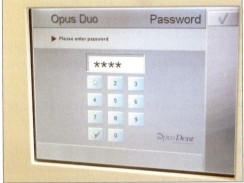
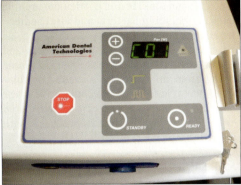
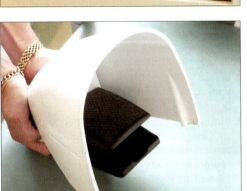
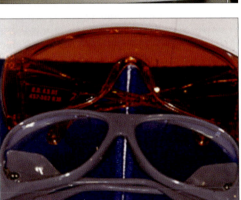

Fig. 12 (left) Password-protected screen

Fig. 13 (right) Key-activated laser, showing 'error code' due to fibre/foot pedal not connected

Fig. 14 (left) Protection for foot pedal

Fig. 15 (right) Laser protection glasses with side-shields

posed by the revised classification are summarised in Figure 1.

The remainder of this chapter will address safety issues associated with Class IV (mainly) and Class III lasers.

RISKS ASSOCIATED WITH LASER USE

Laser beam risks

These risks are those that are posed by exposure of non-target tissues to laser beams. Because of the intensity of the output beam and the ability of lasers to produce very high concentrations of optical power at considerable distances, these lasers can cause serious injuries to the eyes and can also burn the skin.

Optical risks: the majority of laser-induced ocular injuries are considered due to operator error.[16] In general and with specific reference to lasers used in dentistry, there exist two groups of wavelengths that can adversely affect the eye.[17,18] Wavelengths from 400-1,400 nm (visible and near-infrared) can pass through the transparent structures at the front of the eye and impact on the retina (Fig. 2). Longer wavelengths (2,780-10,600 nm, mid- to far-infrared), will interact with the cornea.

In terms of the scope for repair, retinal injuries are more serious.[19-22] Due to the focussing ability of the lens, a 1 mW (0.001 W) laser beam, passing to the back of the eye, results in a retinal irradiance more than 300 W cm^{-2}, well above the ablation threshold. Visible wavelengths may selectively destroy red or green cones, resulting in some colour blindness, although the majority of retinal laser burns affect complete areas of tissue due to the predominance of invisible wavelengths in dental lasers. Retinal injury may initially pass unnoticed, due to the lack of pain receptors.[16]

Longer wavelengths will interact with structures at the front of the eye, causing ablation, scarring and distortion of vision[23] (Fig. 3).

Skin risks: Whilst UV lasers (<400 nm) are not commercially used in dentistry, there is a combined risk of ablative damage to skin structure and possible ionising effects that may be pre-cancerous. All other laser wavelengths can cause 'skin burns'[24,25] due to ablative interaction with target chromophores.

Non-beam risks

These risks are associated with possible physical damage arising from moveable components of a laser, electrical shock and mains supplies (pressurised air, water). Fire risks, through the ignition of tubing, some anaesthetic gases or chemicals (eg alcoholic disinfectants), should be identified and avoided.[26-30] In addition, the products of tissue ablation (plume) represent a considerable hazard that can affect the clinician, auxiliary personnel and the patient. Suitable fine mesh face masks specific to surgical laser use, gloves and high-speed suction aspiration must be used to control the spread of all laser tissue ablation products (see Fig. 4).

Laser plume

Products of laser tissue ablation are collectively termed a 'laser plume'. Whenever non-calcified tissue is ablated, such as in caries removal and all soft tissue surgery, a complex chemical mixture is emitted. This may include water vapour, hydrocarbon gases, carbon monoxide and dioxide and particulate organic material (including bacteria and viral bodies). The effect of plume inhalation can be serious and cause nausea, breathing difficulties and distant inoculation of bacteria.[31-34] The plume arising from mid-infrared wavelength ablation of dental hard tissue is comparatively less potentially dangerous and can be considered similar to the debris that is produced with an air turbine.

LASER SAFETY MEASURES

Within the governing regulations, there exists a need for all specific and stochastic risks to be explored and measures taken to minimise their occurrence. Safety measures applicable to laser use in dental practice can be listed as follows:
- Environment
- Laser protection advisor/laser safety officer
- Access
- Laser safety features
- Eye protection
- Test firing
- Local rules
- Training.

Environment

The concept of laser beam collimation is only true for transmission in a vacuum, or at its immediate exit from the laser cavity. In air, and certainly through a delivery system with or without focussing devices, some divergence will occur. Accepting the power output, amount of divergence and beam diameter and configuration, a nominal ocular hazard distance (NOHD) can be assessed.[35] This is a distance from the laser emission, beyond which the tissue (eye) risk is below the MPE. This is a complex calculation that can be done by a medical physicist, but for a Class IV dental laser, this distance is approximately three metres.

Consequently, as with ionising radiation, the concept of a controlled area can be adopted, within which only those personnel directly involved in laser delivery can enter and with specified protection.[36-39] The controlled area must be delineated with warning signs (Fig. 5) that specify the risk, windows, doors and all surfaces should be non-reflective and access throughways either supervised or operated by remote inter-locks during laser emission. A secure locked designated place for the laser key, if applicable, should be assigned, together with a designated place for all laser accessories. In addition, a suitable fire extinguisher should be sited for easy access.

Safety officers

Dental practices offering Class IIIB and IV laser treatment, must appoint a laser protection advisor (LPA) and a laser safety officer (LSO). The LPA is usually a medical physicist who will advise on the protective devices required, MPE and NOHD for any given laser wavelength being used. The LSO is appointed to ensure that all safety aspects of laser use are identified and enforced. Ideally, this could be a suitably trained and qualified dental surgery assistant. Duties of the LSO include the following:
- Confirm classification of the laser
- Read manufacturers' instructions concerning installation, use and maintenance of the laser equipment
- Make sure that laser equipment is properly assembled for use
- Train workers in safe use of lasers
- Oversee controlled area and limit access
- Oversee maintenance protocols for laser equipment
- Post appropriate warning signs
- Recommend appropriate personal protective equipment such as eye wear and protective clothing
- Maintain a log of all laser procedures carried out, relative to each patient, the procedure and laser operating parameters
- Maintain an adverse effects reporting system
- Assume overall control for laser use and interrupt treatment if any safety measure is infringed.

Access

Relative to, for example, a hospital operating theatre, most dental surgeries exist within rooms with physical barriers – walls and one or possibly two access doors. As such, non-authorised access can be controlled easily. However, most Class IV lasers have a remote inter-lock jack socket, whereby door locks and warning lights can be activated during laser emission. Those dental clinics that operate a multi-chair, open-plan environment would need to address the requirement in greater detail. During laser treatment, only the clinician, assistant and patient should be allowed within the controlled area.

Laser safety features

All lasers have in-built safety features that must be cross-matched to allow laser emission (Figs 6-14). These include:
- Emergency 'Stop' button
- Emission port shutters to prevent laser emission until the correct delivery system is attached
- Covered foot-switch, to prevent accidental operation
- Control panel to ensure correct emission parameters
- Audible or visual signs of laser emission
- Locked unit panels to prevent unauthorised access to internal machinery
- Key or password protection
- Remote inter-locks.

Eye protection

All persons within the controlled area must wear appropriate eye protection during laser

REGULATION

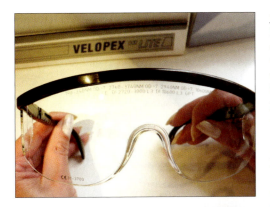

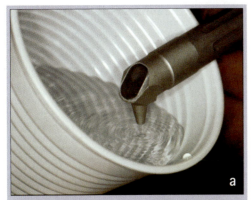

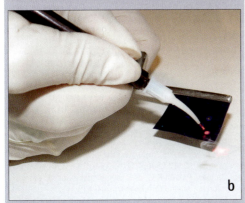

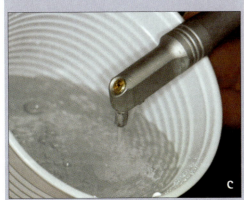

emission. It is considered advisable to cover the patient's eyes with damp gauze for long wavelength peri-oral procedures.[40] The LSO should select the correct eyewear for the laser wavelength being used, these should free of any scratches or damage and be constructed with side protection (Figs 15 and 16).

Such eye protection must then be properly specified for the exposure conditions that could occur, and its use must be subject to a strictly-enforced written policy. In Europe, laser eye protection must conform to either EN 207 or EN 208, and be CE marked to indicate compliance with European legislation. All protection glasses or goggles should be marked with the wavelength for which protection is given, together with a value of optical density (OD).[41] The OD refers to the ability of a material to reduce laser energy of a specific wavelength to a safe level below the MPE. The OD value should be '5.0' or above for adequate protection. In addition, through the new regulation, other factors are now deemed necessary and these are listed as follows:

- Requirements under ANSI Z 136 (USA): OD values >5 to ensure attenuation to MPE values
- Requirements under EN207/208/60825: direct impact (DIN) values >5. Under this directive, protective eyewear should be able to attenuate direct beam exposure to MPE values within the following parameters: 10 seconds (continuous wave (CW) emission) and 100 pulses (free-running pulsed emission)
- Requirements under ANSI & EN 207: protective laser eyewear should carry specific labelling to define: OD, optical density; DIR operation mode; wavelength (nm); L6A protective grade; RH manufacturer's mark; DIN testing standard; CE (applicable for European distribution).

The L6A protective grade defines the suitability for the eyewear within clinical, industrial or research conditions. OD and DIN values should be >5.0. Wavelength values may be specific, eg 400 nm, or grouped, eg 2,780-10,600 nm. 'DIR' defines the operation (emission) mode of the laser. Each value is measured against the following coding: 'D' = CW mode, 'I' = pulsed mode, 'R' = Q-switched mode.

An example of what should appear on a pair of correctly prescribed Nd:YAG protective glasses is as follows: OD5/ IR 1064nm/ L6A/ RH/ DIN5 (+CE).

Test firing

Prior to any laser procedure and before admitting the patient, either the clinician or LSO should test-fire the laser. This is to establish that the laser has been assembled correctly, is working correctly and that laser emission is occurring through the delivery system. Protective eyewear is worn and all other safety measures met. The laser is directed towards a suitable absorbent material, eg water for long wavelengths and dark coloured paper for short wavelengths, and operated at the lowest power setting for the laser being used (Fig. 17). Following this, the laser is inactivated and the patient admitted.

Local rules

As with ionising radiation, a set of local rules must be compiled for practices carrying out

Fig. 16 CE mark and OD values for wavelength protection (>5.0)

Fig. 17 Test firing procedures for CO_2 (a), diode (b) and Er:YAG (c) lasers. Low-power settings and suitable attenuation materials (water and dark paper) allow pre-treatment checks as to correct laser function and patency of delivery systems

laser treatment. The LPA can help with drawing up this document, but it should include the following:
- Name and address of the practice
- Each laser used, identified by manufacturer, wavelength, emission mode, power output, delivery system and serial number
- Personnel permitted to use the laser
- Designation of the authority and responsibility for the evaluation and control of laser hazards to a laser safety officer
- A written laser safety policy, to include all safety aspects of laser use
- Establishment of a quality assurance program including regular inspection and maintenance of the laser equipment
- Training and education of personnel involved in the use of lasers
- Management of incidents and accidents, including reporting, investigation, analysis and remedial action.

The local rules should be read and signed by all practice personnel involved in delivery of laser treatment and should be updated regularly.

Training

All staff members should receive objective and recognised training in the safety aspects of laser use within dentistry, as with other specialties.[42-44] There is no legal obligation for this, although the Healthcare Commission would consider this to be part of the national minimal standards, against which the registered practice is inspected. National bodies, such as the National Physics Laboratory and the NRPB, offer courses in laser safety, although dental laser organisations such as ESOLA and the ALD carry examination-based LSO grading courses.

CONCLUSION

The consequence of excess laser power delivered to target tissue has been presented in previous chapters in this book. Above a range of maximum permitted exposure values, non-target tissue is subject to accidental exposure which, in the case of the eye, can result in permanent damage. Anyone working with or responsible for potentially hazardous laser equipment should be properly trained in laser safety, be aware of the nature of laser hazards and understand the procedures and safeguards that need to be implemented. Employers have to establish an adequate safety policy for the management and control of risks arising from the use of laser equipment.

The current legal framework for laser safety is a somewhat blurred overlap of competing regulations, but a 'best practice' approach to laser safety, often to address a 'worst case' scenario, is essential. The classification of lasers defines power capability relative to ocular risk, protective eyewear is specified to attenuate laser light within dedicated individual limits and the general approach to laser safety within the workplace serves to protect the patient and staff.

1. Statutory Instrument 2004 No.664. *The health and social care (community health and standards) act 2003 (commission for healthcare audit and inspection and commission for social care inspection) (transitional and consequential provisions) order 2004*. London: The Stationery Office, 2004.
2. Sliney D H. Evolving issues in laser safety. *J Laser Appl* 1997; **9:** 295-300.
3. Source: UK Health Protection Agency, 2005.
4. International Electrotechnical Commission. *Safety of laser products – part 1: equipment classification, requirements, and user's guide*. IEC 60825-1/A2:2001. Geneva: IEC, 1993; with amendment 2, 2001.
5. European Committee for Electrotechnical Standardization. *Safety of laser products – part 1: equipment classification, requirements, and user's guide*. Brussels: European Committee for Electrotechnical Standardization, 1994; with amendment 2, 2001.
6. Health and social care (community health and standards) act 2003. Chapter 43 explanatory notes. London: The Stationery Office, 2003.
7. *Safety of laser products – part 14: a user's guide*. PD IEC TR 60825-14:2004. British Standards, 2004.
8. Takac S, Stojanovic S. Classification of laser irradiation and safety measures. *Med Pregl* 1998; **51:** 415-418.
9. Sliney D, Aron-Rosa D, DeLori F et al. Adjustment of guidelines for exposure of the eye to optical radiation from ocular instruments: statement from a task group of the International Commission on Non-Ionizing Radiation Protection (ICNIRP). *Appl Opt* 2005; **44:** 2162-2176.
10. International Electrotechnical Commission. *Safety of laser products – part 9: compilation of maximum permissible exposure to incoherent radiation*. IEC TR 60825-9: 1999-10. Geneva: IEC, 1999.
11. Sethi C S, Grey R H, Hart C D. Laser pointers revisited: a survey of 14 patients attending casualty at the Bristol Eye Hospital. *Br J Ophthalmol* 1999; **83:** 1164-1167.
12. Robertson D M, McLaren J W, Salomao D R, Link T P. Retinopathy from a green laser pointer: a clinicopathologic study. *Arch Ophthalmol* 2005; **123:** 629-633.
13. Reidenbach H D, Dollinger K, Hofmann J. Field trials with low power lasers concerning the blink reflex. *Biomed Tech (Berl)* 2002; **47 (Suppl 1):** 600-601.
14. Chandra P, Azad R V. Laser rangefinder induced retinal injuries. *Indian J Ophthalmol* 2004; **52:** 349.
15. Schuele G, Rumohr M, Huettmann G, Brinkmann R. RPE damage thresholds and mechanisms for laser exposure in the microsecond-to-millisecond time regimen. *Invest Ophthalmol Vis Sci* 2005; **46:** 714-719.
16. Moseley H. Operator error is the key factor contributing to medical laser accidents. *Lasers Med Sci* 2004; **19:** 105-111.
17. Barkana Y, Belkin M. Laser eye injuries. *Surv Ophthalmol* 2000; **44:** 459-478.
18. Thach A B. Laser injuries of the eye. *Int Ophthalmol Clin* 1999; **39(2):** 13-27.
19. Hagemann L F, Costa R A, Ferreira H M, Farah M E. Optical coherence tomography of a traumatic neodymium:YAG laser-induced macular hole. *Ophthalmic Surg Lasers Imaging* 2003; **34:** 57-59.
20. Chuang L H, Lai C C, Yang K J, Chen T L, Ku W C. A traumatic macular hole secondary to a high-energy Nd:YAG laser. *Ophthalmic Surg Lasers* 2001; **32:** 73-76.
21. Clarke T F, Johnson T E, Burton M B, Ketzenberger B, Roach W P. Corneal injury threshold in rabbits for the 1540 nm infrared laser. *Aviat Space Environ Med* 2002; **73:** 787-790.
22. Harris M D, Lincoln A E, Amoroso P J, Stuck B, Sliney D. Laser eye injuries in military occupations. *Aviat Space Environ Med* 2003; **74:** 947-952.
23. Widder R A, Severin M, Kirchhof B, Krieglstein G K. Corneal injury after carbon dioxide laser skin resurfacing. *Am J Ophthalmol* 1998; **125:** 392-394.
24. Miedziak A I, Gottsch J D, Iliff N T. Exposure keratopathy after cosmetic CO_2 laser skin resurfacing. *Cornea* 2000; **19:** 846-848.
25. Grossman A R, Majidian A M, Grossman P H. Thermal injuries as a result of CO_2 laser resurfacing. *Plast Reconstr Surg* 1998; **102:** 1247-1252.

REGULATION

26. Ilgner J, Falter F, Westhofen M. Long-term follow-up after laser-induced endotracheal fire. *J Laryngol Otol* 2002; **116:** 213-215.
27. Macdonald A G. A brief historical review of non-anaesthetic causes of fires and explosions in the operating room. *Br J Anaesth* 1994; **73:** 847-856.
28. Sosis M B, Braverman B. Evaluation of foil coverings for protecting plastic endotracheal tubes from the potassium-titanyl-phosphate laser. *Anesth Analg* 1993; **77:** 589-591.
29. Cork R C. Anesthesia for otolaryngologic surgery involving use of a laser. *Contemp Anesth Pract* 1987; **9:** 127-140.
30. Dave R, Mahaffey P J. The control of fire hazard during cutaneous laser therapy. *Lasers Med Sci* 2002; **17:** 6-8.
31. Scott E, Beswick A, Wakefield K. The hazards of diathermy plume. Part 2. Producing quantified data. *Br J Perioper Nurs* 2004; **14:** 452, 454-456.
32. Garden J M, O'Banion M K, Bakus A D, Olson C. Viral disease transmitted by laser-generated plume (aerosol). *Arch Dermatol* 2002; **138:** 1303-1307.
33. Kunachak S, Sobhon P. The potential alveolar hazard of carbon dioxide laser-induced smoke. *J Med Assoc Thai* 1998; **81:** 278-282.
34. McKinley I B Jr, Ludlow M O. Hazards of laser smoke during endodontic therapy. *J Endod* 1994; **20:** 558-559.
35. Sterenborg H J. Lasers in dentistry. 9. Safety in laser use. *Ned Tijdschr Tandheelkd* 2003; **110:** 62-66.
36. Andersen K. Safe use of lasers in the operating room – what perioperative nurses should know. *AORN J* 2004; **79:** 171-88.
37. Marshall W J, Aldrich R C, Zimmerman S A. Laser hazard evaluation method for middle infrared laser systems. *J Laser Appl* 1996; **8:** 211-216.
38. Schmidt F U. Ophthalmological risks and hazards of laser use in the head and neck region. *Adv Otorhinolaryngol* 1995; **49:** 23-26.
39. Szymanska J. Work-related vision hazards in the dental office. *Ann Agric Environ Med* 2000; **7:** 1-4.
40. Bhattacharyya N, Richard C. A comparison of ocular protective measures during carbon dioxide laser laryngoscopy. *Arch Otolaryngol Head Neck Surg* 2004; **130:** 1289-1292.
41. Laser safety eyewear. *Health Devices* 1993; **22:** 159-204.
42. Youker S R, Ammirati C T. Practical aspects of laser safety. *Facial Plast Surg* 2001; **17:** 155-163.
43. Lewandowski M A, Hinz M W. A simple approach to industrial laser safety. Health Phys 2005; **88 (Suppl 2):** S24-S30.
44. Edwards B E, Barnes L K, Gibbs J B, Nguyen G B. Medical laser safety hazard evaluation. Health Phys 2002; **83 (Suppl 8):** S36-S44.

LASERS IN DENTISTRY

Absorption 13-15
  pigmented versus non-pigmented tissues 16
  secondary factors 16-17
Absorption coefficients 13, 16
Access, safety measures 76
Actinobacillus actinomycetemcomitans 47
Active medium 7
  energy exchange 9-10
Air embolism 66
Analgesic effects
  low-level laser therapy 22
  pulpal 64
Aphthous ulceration 23
Applications 1
Argon ion laser 3, 4
  composite resin curing 24
  dental use 4
Arndt Schultz law 22
Articulated arm delivery systems 8, 17

Back-scatter 12
Bacterial contamination, surgical incision-related 29
  avoidance with laser surgery 31, 36
Bacterial decontamination 1, 19
  endodontics 53, 54-55
  peri-implantitis 52-53
  periodontal therapy 43, 47
Bacteroides forsythus 47
Beam
  dynamics 10
  exposure risks 74
  movement for thermal relaxation 15
Biostimulation see Photobiostimulation
Blood flow, thermal relaxation effect 15
Blood spatter exposure 66
Bone ablation 19, 47
  erbium lasers 65-66
BS EN 60825-1:1994 72

Calculus removal 43, 47
Camphorquinone 24
Carbon dioxide laser 3, 4
  active medium 9
  energy exchange 9-10
  hard tissue interactions 18, 19, 60
  implant placement studies 52
  periodontal therapy 45
  pulp capping 54
  root canal
    access/shaping 54
    bacterial decontamination 54-55
  soft tissue surgery 31, 37
  'laser peel' of flat lesions 35
  target tissue absorption 16, 36
Care Standards Act (2000) 70, 73
Caries detection 1
  low-level lasers 24-26
  polarisation-sensitive optical coherence tomography (PS-OCT) 25-26
  quantitative light-induced fluorescence 24, 25
  safety 74
Carious tissue ablation 19, 62
Cavities, laser scanning 27

Cavity preparation 19, 60, 62-63
  erbium lasers 19
    dentine 65
    enamel 64-65
    pain perception 64
    pulpal temperature rise 63
CE markings 72
Cementum, erbium laser ablation 19
Chopped continuous wave emission mode 10
Chromophores 16
Class I lasers 74
Class II lasers 74
Class III lasers 74
  safety 76
Class IV lasers 74
  safety 76
Classification of lasers, regulatory aspects 73-75
Co-axial water spray 19, 61, 65, 66
Coagulum layer 18, 31
Collimation 7, 10, 76
Composite resin curing 1, 24
Continuous wave mode 10, 15, 51
Contolled areas 76
Control panel 8, 10
Cooling system 8, 15
  co-axial water spray 19, 61, 65, 66

Delivery systems 8, 17
  endodontics 54
  periodontal therapy 44-45
Dentine ablation 18, 19, 61, 62
  erbium laser cavity preparation 65
Dentine hypersensitivity 55-56
  low-level laser therapy 23
Denture granuloma 31, 35
Diode lasers 8-9
  back-scatter 12
  dentine hypersensitivity treatment 55
  implants
    peri-implantitis 52
    placement studies 51
    soft tissue management 52
  periodontal therapy 45, 47
    with methylene blue 47
  photobiostimulation 21
  root canal bacterial decontamination 54, 55
  soft tissue surgery 31, 35, 37
  target tissue absorption 16, 36
Dressings 29, 36

Electric shock 75
Emission mode 10
  laser light absorption influence 16
Enamel ablation 18, 19, 61, 62
  erbium laser cavity preparation 64-65
Endodontics 53-57
  bacterial decontamination 26, 53, 54-55
  gutta percha material sealing/removal 55
Energy exchange 9-10
  peak power discharge 10
Enterococcus faecalis 26, 55
Environmental safety measures 76
Epulis 36, 38

Er:YAG laser 5, 7, 10
  cavity preparation
    enamel 65
    pain perception 64
  hard tissues cutting 18, 19, 61
  peri-implantitis 52
  periodontal therapy 44, 45, 47
  photoplasmolysis 14
  root canal access/shaping 54
  soft tissue surgery 31, 35
    combined hard tissue treatment 38
  target tissue absorption 16, 36
Erbium lasers 7
  bone ablation 19, 47, 65-66
  calculus removal 47
  cavity preparation 64-65
    dentine 65
    enamel 64-65
    pain perception 64
  cementum ablation 19
  dentine hypersensitivity 56
  hand-pieces 62
  hard tissue cutting 18-19, 61-62
  implants
    placement applications 50, 52
    soft tissue management 52
  root dentine ablation 19
Er,Cr:YSGG laser 5, 7
  hard tissues cutting 18, 19, 61
  peri-implantitis 52
  periodontal therapy 44, 45, 47
  root canal
    access/shaping 54
    bacterial decontamination 55
  soft tissue surgery 31, 34
    combined hard tissue treatment 38
  target tissue absorption 16, 36
Escherichia coli 55
European Community directives 72
  eye protection 77
European Standard EN 60825-1 72, 74
Exposure time, absorption influence 16
Extra-oral muscle groups, low-level laser fluence 23
Eyes
  exposure risk 74, 75, 78
  protection 66, 71, 73, 74, 76-77

Facial swellings, laser scanning 27
Factor VII 18
Fibroma 31
Fire risk 74, 75
Flashes 14
Fluence (energy density)
  low-level lasers 23
  surgical/cutting lasers 23
Fluoridated enamel ablation 64
Four-level energy exchange 9-10
Fraenectomy 31, 35
Free-running pulsed mode 10
  gingival surgery 38
  implant placement studies 51, 52
  peak power levels 10, 11, 23
    hard tissue cutting 18-19
  thermal relaxation 15
Frequency-doubled alexandrite, calculus

INDEX

removal 44, 47
Fusobacterium nucleatum 26

Gated emission 10
Gaussian beam 10
Giant cell granuloma 36, 37
Gingival hyperplasia 36, 38
   drug-induced 38
   orthodontic appliances-related 38
Gingival tissue
   implant margins 52
   laser interactions 36-37
   low-level laser fluence (energy density) 23
Gutta percha sealing/removal 55

Haemangioma 31
Haemoglobin 16
Haemostasis 1, 18, 19, 36
   endodontics 54
   periodontal therapy 43, 45
   soft tissue laser surgery 31, 35
Hand-piece delivery systems 8, 62
   'laser drill' development 62
   periodontal therapy 45
      calculus removal 47
Hard (surgical) lasers 12
Hard tissues 1, 60-68
   'laser drill' development 60-63
   laser interactions 18-19
      beneficial aspects 19
Healthcare Commission 70, 71, 73
Herpes labialis 23
Herpes simplex 23
Historical aspects 1, 2-3
   dental use 4-5
   medical/surgical use 3-4
Ho:YAG laser 7
Hollow waveguide delivery system 8, 17, 45
Holmium lasers 7
Hydrokinetic effect 61
Hydroxyapatite 16, 18, 64
   post-laser characteristics 60

IEC 60825-1 72
Implantology 50-53
   implant placement studies 50-52
   peri-implantitis 52-53
   soft tissue management 52
Incident angle of beam, absorption influence 16
International Electro-technical Commission (IEC) recommendations 72, 73

Keratinised mucosa-laser interactions 36-37
KTP laser, periodontal therapy 43

Labelling of lasers, regulations 73
Labial fraenectomy 31
'Laser drill' 60-63
Laser light 3, 7
   beam dynamics 10
   emission modes 10
   wavelength *see* Wavelength, laser

Laser pointers 74
Laser safety officer 70, 76, 77, 78
Laser scanning 27
Laser-ENAP (excisional new attachment procedure) 43, 45
Laser-tissue interactions 12-20
   beneficial aspects 19
   hard tissues 19
   soft tissues 19, 36-37
Lasers
   classification 73-75
   component parts 7-8
      active medium 7
      control panel 8
      cooling system 8
      delivery system 8
      optical resonator 8
      pumping mechanism 7-8
   four-level energy exchange 9-10
   low-level *see* Low-level lasers
   regulatory standards 72
   safety features 76
   test firing 77
Legal aspects 72-73
Lichen planus, non-erosive 31, 35
Light
   absorption/emission 5-7
   ordinary 5
   photonic energy 5
   quantum nature 5-7
   see also Laser light
Lingual fraenectomy 31, 35
Local rules 77-78
Low-level lasers 21-27
   caries detection 24-26
   clinical applications 23
   composite resin curing 24
   dosimetry 22
   fluence (energy density) 23
   laser units 22-23
   photo-activated disinfection 26
   photobiostimulation 22
   safety regulations 74
   scanning 27

Maser 3
Maximal average power output 10
Maximal permissible exposure (MPE) 74, 76
Melanin 16, 36
   patches ablation 41
Metal vapour laser 3
Methylene blue chemical mediator 47
Minimally-invasive restorations 19
Mucocoele 31
Mucocytosis 31

Nd:YAG laser 3, 4, 5, 7
   back-scatter 12
   dental use 4
   dentine hypersensitivity 55-56
   hard tissue interactions 18, 60
   implants
      placement studies 50, 51, 52
      soft tissue management 52
   periodontal therapy 45

laser-ENAP 43, 45
photoplasmolysis 14
pulp capping 54
pulpal analgesia 64
root canal
   access/shaping 54
      bacterial decontamination 54
soft tissue surgery 31
target tissue absorption 16, 36
thermal damage risk 37
Neuropathy 23
Nominal ocular hazard distance (NOHD) 76

Oedema prevention 19, 31
Optical resonator 8
Oral epithelium, low-level laser fluence 23
Oral infections 26
Oral swellings, laser scanning 27
Orthodontics 38
   brackets placement 38, 63
   laser scanning 27
Osteotomy site preparation 50

Pain perception
   cavity preparation 64
   see also Analgesic effects
Patient experience 1
Peak power capacity 10, 11, 16
   free-running pulsed mode 10, 11, 23
      hard tissue cutting 18-19
Peptostreptococcus micros 26
Peri-implantitis 52-53
Periodontal therapy 43-48
   calculus removal 43, 47
   laser wavelengths 43, 44
   pocket epithelium bacterial decontamination 43, 44-47
   risk analysis 44
   sub-gingival curettage 45
Photo-activated disinfection 26
Photobiostimulation 12, 13, 21-22, 56
   analgesic effects 22
   clinical acceptance 23
   clinical applications 23
   laser units 22-23
   low-level laser therapy 21-22
   stimulatory effects 22
Photoelectric effect 2
Photon 5
Photonic emission, stimulated 5
Photoplasmolysis 14-15
Photopyrolysis 14
Photothermal effects 12, 13
Photothermolysis 14, 37
Photovaporolysis 14
Plasma formation 10, 14-15
Plume inhalation risks 75-76
Polarisation-sensitive optical coherence tomography (PS-OCT) 25-26
Popping sounds, hard tissue interactions 14, 61
Porphyromonas gingivalis 47
Post-extraction socket 23
Post-oncology disorders 23
Post-trauma sites 23
Prevotella intermedia 26, 47

Pulp capping 53-54
Pulpal analgesia 64
Pulpal temperature rise 18, 19, 24, 60
  during cavity preparation 63
Pulpotomy 53-54
Pulsed dye lasers 4
Pulsed erbium lasers 5
Pulsed wave mode 10, 51
  target tissue thermal relaxation 10, 11, 15
Pumping mechanism 7-8

Q-switched emission mode 10
Quantitative light-induced fluorescence, caries detection 24, 25
Quartz optic fibre delivery system 8, 17
  endodontic applications 54
  periodontal therapy 44

Raman spectroscopy 27
Reflection 12-13
Registration of practitioners 70-73
Regulations 70-73
  laser classification 73-75
Root canal therapy 53
  access/shaping of canal walls 54
  thermal damage risk 54
Root dentine
  desensitisation 53
  erbium laser ablation 19
Ruby laser 3, 4

Safety
  Class I lasers 74
  Class II lasers 74
  Class III lasers 74
  Class IV lasers 74
  laser beam risks 74, 75
  laser plume inhalation 75-76
  legislation 72
  non-beam risks 75
  ocular risk 74, 75, 78
  regulatory requirements 70, 71
  skin exposure risk 74, 75
Safety measures 76-78
  access 76
  environment 76
  equipment 76
    standards 72
  eye protection 76-77
  laser safety officers 76
  local rules 77-78
  test firing 77
  training 78
Sapphire hand-piece tips 45
Scanning, laser 27
Scar formation 29, 31
Scatter 12
Secondary intention healing 18, 29
Skin exposure risks 74, 75
'Soft' lasers 12
  safety regulations 74
Soft tissues
  implant site management 52
  laser interactions 17-18
    beneficial aspects 19
    keratinised mucosa 36-37
  laser surgery 29-35, 36-41
    benign pathology excision 37-41
    combined hard tissue treatment 38
    gingival cuff preservation 36
    pre-treatment gingival assessment 36-37
    protective coagulum formation 18, 31
    surgical procedure 31, 34-35
    thermal damage risk 31, 34-35, 36, 37
    wound healing 29
    post-incisional bacterial contamination 29, 31, 36
Sterilisation effect 19
  see also Bacterial decontamination
Streptococcus intermedius 26
Streptococcus mutans 26
Super-pulsed emission mode 10
Surface wetting, absorption influence 16
Sutures 29, 35, 36

Temporomandibular joint disorders 23
Test firing 77
Thermal relaxation 10, 11, 15, 16
  soft tissue laser surgery 31, 34, 35, 37-38
Tissue composition/thickness, absorption influence 16
Titanium reflectivity 51, 52
Tooth fracture/fracture margin exposure 36, 38
Training 70, 71, 74, 78
Transmission 12
Transverse electromagnetic modes 10
Treponema denticola 47
Treponema sokranskii 47
Trigeminal neuralgia 23

Unerupted tooth exposure 38
USA
  eye protection standards 77
  laser classification 73
  regulatory requirements 72

Water 16
  dental hard tissues 18
    erbium laser cavity preparation 64, 65
    'laser drill' development 61-62
Water spray 19, 52, 61, 65, 66
Waveguide delivery system 8, 17
  periodontal therapy 45
Wavelength, laser 7
  endodontics 53, 54
  hard tissue interactions 18, 60-61
    cutting dynamics 18-19
  'laser drill' development 60
  periodontal therapy 43, 44
  photonic energy relationship 5
  soft tissue surgery 18, 31, 36-37
  target tissue absorption influence 16
Wound healing 1, 29
  implant soft tissues 52
  lased bone 66
  secondary intention 18, 29